Reflections of a Microvascular Plastic Surgeon

This book discusses the scope and limitations of complex reconstructive surgery that few plastic surgeons master, and that the public rarely encounters, portraying both the technical challenges of advanced reconstructive microsurgery and the human connection between physician and patient as only a master surgeon can convey.

For decades, Dr. Deleyiannis has practiced one of the most demanding fields of surgery, treating patients with highly complex and devastating deformities from cancer, trauma, and birth anomalies. Laying the historical foundation of scientific discoveries upon which modern microsurgical practice is based, he takes us "behind the scenes" with real patients' stories, highlighting surgical innovation in his own career and the impact on the lives of those he treats.

Plastic surgeons and surgeons specializing in reconstruction techniques for patients who have suffered either trauma or cancer will find inspiration and renewed dedication for their specialism within the pages of this book.

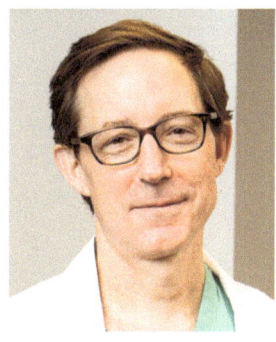

Frederic White-Brown Deleyiannis MD, MPhil, MPH, FACS

Dr. Deleyiannis is a board-certified surgeon in both Plastic Surgery and Otolaryngology – Head and Neck Surgery. He is a graduate of the University of Pennsylvania, Yale School of Medicine, and the University of Cambridge, England. His practice for over 20 years has focused on providing the clinical care, leadership, and education to treat the most complex reconstructive cases after cancer and trauma. He is the author or coauthor of over 100 published peer-reviewed articles and book chapters in major medical journals and textbooks. Previously, he was Associate Professor at the University of Pittsburgh and Professor of Surgery at the University of Colorado. Presently, he is the Medical Practice Leader of Plastic Surgery and Director of Microvascular Surgery for UCHealth in Colorado Springs, Colorado.

ADVANCED PRAISE

Dr. Deleyiannis poignantly portrays both the technical challenges of advanced reconstructive microsurgery and the human connection between physician and patient as only a master surgeon can convey.

J. Peter Rubin, MD, MBA, UPMC *Endowed Professor and Chair, Department of Plastic Surgery, University of Pittsburgh, Past President, American Society of Plastic Surgeons*

Here is a look at the careful evaluation, planning, and expert performance to save life and limb of a fellow human being. A tale of technical expertise and modern medicine, it is a view of intense, driving humanity.

Ernest K. Manders, MD, *Professor Emeritus, Department of Plastic Surgery, University of Pittsburgh School of Medicine*

The unique and vital approach to reconstruction with its concise narrative and detailed imagery will serve as a well-used reference for surgeons considering this career trajectory, those already practicing microvascular reconstructive surgery, and patients and their families.

Neal Futran, MD, DMD, *Allison Wannamaker Professor and Chair, Director of Head and Neck Surgery, Department of Otolaryngology-HNS, University of Washington*

Reflections of a Microvascular Plastic Surgeon

Reconstructing Shattered Lives

Frederic White-Brown Deleyiannis

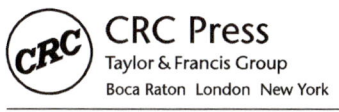

CRC Press
Taylor & Francis Group
Boca Raton London New York

CRC Press is an imprint of the
Taylor & Francis Group, an **informa** business

First edition published 2025
by CRC Press
2385 NW Executive Center Drive, Suite 320, Boca Raton FL 33431

and by CRC Press
4 Park Square, Milton Park, Abingdon, Oxon, OX14 4RN

CRC Press is an imprint of Taylor & Francis Group, LLC

ISBN: 978-1-032-88485-1 (hbk)
ISBN: 978-1-032-81742-2 (pbk)
ISBN: 978-1-003-53802-8 (ebk)

DOI: 10.1201/9781003538028

Typeset in Sabon
by SPi Technologies India Pvt Ltd (Straive)

For my loving parents, Mary and Steve Deleyiannis, who gave me the gifts of an education and a strong work ethic.

To my wife, Anna, and my daughters, Paloma and Leonor, who inspire me to put those gifts in the service of a meaningful purpose.

Contents

Author's Note

The stories here of patients are all real. To protect confidentiality, I have changed some patient names and minor identifying details. Whenever such changes were made, I have documented these changes in the text. Prior to publication, all of the patients and their families gave consent to have their stories told and allowed photographs and figures to be used. Their edits and comments were incorporated into the final manuscript. Regional and/or national press have also covered and personally interviewed some of the patients and their families. These interviews and publications are documented in the respective chapters. One of the challenges of writing a book about microsurgery is how to demonstrate the complexity of the procedures. To provide visual explanations, surgical diagrams have been included. With the exception of those figures directly referenced, all surgical diagrams were illustrated by Kelly Li (Harvard Medical School, Class of 2026).

Foreword I

Eugene N. Myers

Frederic White-Brown Deleyiannis has been a leader in plastic surgery for more than 20 years. He is a graduate of the University of Pennsylvania. He received his MD from Yale, followed by a residency in otolaryngology at the University of Washington, a fellowship in microvascular and head and neck surgery in Oviedo, Spain, and a second residency in plastic surgery at the University of Pittsburgh. It was there that I met him. I was Chairman of the Department of Otolaryngology and had a robust practice in surgery of the head and neck and interacted with Fred who was outstanding in the micro-surgical reconstruction of the extensive surgical defects that I produced.

After advancing to an Associate Professor, he moved on and ultimately became Professor of Plastic Surgery at the University of Colorado and Chief of Pediatric Plastic Surgery at the Children's Hospital Colorado. Presently, Fred is the Medical Practice Leader of Plastic Surgery at UCHealth Memorial Hospital in Colorado Springs, one of the busiest Level I trauma centers in Colorado. He is a nationally recognized expert in microvascular surgery, particularly free tissue transfer. He specializes in operating on patients with complex trauma and reconstruction following cancer surgery. Fred is also a trained epidemiologist and statistician whose ongoing research focuses on the effectiveness of different types of reconstruction for patients undergoing these surgeries.

The book is a pleasure to read as one would expect from an author who also has a master of philosophy in the history of medicine from the University of Cambridge. As I read the book, I was always aware that the dominant theme was quality of life following microsurgery. Included in his book are details of the preoperative evaluation of the patient, the surgical procedure, postoperative recovery, and long-term follow-up. Fred explains his unique style of preparing his frightened patients by providing compassionate and sensitive care and quietly instilling confidence and trust to proceed with surgery knowing that he has the skill set and expertise to back this up.

There are no books yet like this in academics or in the medical litera-ture because it is much more than just a surgical atlas of operations. Dr. Deleyiannis's low-key style offers a unique look into the life of a microvascular surgeon and should be read by anyone planning to enter this field. In addition to offering a historical perspective of microsurgery, it shows in a very real sense what it is like to be a modern microsurgeon from a standpoint of dedication, work-life balance, opportunity cost, and expertise. I believe anyone interested in microsurgery, in particular plastic surgeons and otolaryngologists, would benefit from reading this book. The audience for the book is also meant to include other doctors who may be involved in cancer and/or trauma care, and patients or families who wish to see what is beyond the "routine explanation" for reconstruction that has been or will be recommended.

Dr. Deleyiannis's main goal was to produce a book that clearly captures the complexity and clinical importance of microsurgery. He achieves this goal. I expect this book will inspire others to enter the specialty and prove to be a valuable resource for doctors and patients alike.

Eugene N. Myers MD, FACS, FRCS, Edin (Hon)
Emeritus Distinguished Professor and Chairman,
Department of Otolaryngology – Head and Neck Surgery
Director, International Visiting Scholars Program

Foreword II

Neal Futran

When one thinks about head and neck reconstruction, the influence and importance of Dr. Frederic White-Brown Deleyiannis cannot be underestimated. With his unique training in both otolaryngology – head and neck surgery – and plastic and reconstructive surgery, he is uniquely prepared to advance this field.

Dr. Deleyiannis's approach to the reconstruction of the most challenging oncologic and traumatic defects, as well as the functional rehabilitation of the patient, has contributed to the rapid evolution of our ability to make our patients "whole". A major portion of *Reflections of a Microvascular Plastic Surgeon: Reconstructing Shattered Lives* stresses the tissue aspects of the reconstruction, carefully assessing thickness, pliability, reliability, color match, donor defect, functional benefits, and side effects of every choice. This can often necessitate a more difficult reconstruction but ultimately benefits the patient. Not only are a broad repertoire of donor sites and techniques necessary, but the surgeon must possess skill and creativity to optimize results in every case. It is equally important to follow and critically evaluate surgical and functional results to consistently improve outcomes. Dr. Deleyiannis also places critical emphasis on patient quality of life and the patient journey and provides essential "takeaways" for patients and families to help them in their journey.

The unique and vital approach to reconstruction with its concise narrative and detailed imagery will serve as a well-used reference for surgeons considering this career trajectory, those already practicing microvascular reconstructive surgery, and also patients and their families. Most importantly, it will help provide better and lifelong outcomes for patients requiring complex reconstruction.

Neal Futran, MD, DMD
Allison Wannamaker Professor and Chair
Director of Head and Neck Surgery
Department of Otolaryngology-HNS
University of Washington

Introduction

This book discusses the scope and limitations of plastic surgery, in particular concerning the most complex reconstructive surgery that few plastic surgeons master and that the public rarely encounters unless he/she suffers a terrible trauma or cancer. This is not the plastic surgery that is glorified in the media by makeovers, remedies for "botched surgery", or blogs about the best breast implant, or that which advertises how one can rejuvenate or refresh oneself with cosmetic procedures or facial fillers. This surgery reimburses the surgeon, not necessarily with the financial gain of cosmetic surgery, but more importantly with the quiet awareness that he has just helped someone recover from a life-altering event.

Why would a plastic surgeon write such a book? In addition to increasing public awareness about the availability of such services, it also serves as a way to search for some meaning in the performance of that surgery. It is a meaning that extends beyond the technical challenges of working with your hands. Who can gaze upon a body destroyed by cancer or trauma and not feel empathy and question how one defines their future? Why are some patients crushed by their disease though they have been cured of it and "successfully reconstructed", while others enter the next chapter of their life with new meaning and purpose?

To be able to provide the highest level of reconstructive plastic surgery, one must be fully trained and devoted to the field of microvascular surgery. Microvascular surgery is the practice of transferring one part of the body, one piece of flesh, with a blood supply that you first disconnect from another part of the body and then reconnect at the site of the injury. It is transplant surgery, but within your own body and with much smaller blood vessels that need to be sewn together under the microscope. Depending on the complexity, microsurgical operations take 5–8 hours, and sometimes 10–20 hours. For the surgeon, each operation can be a test of both physical and mental stamina.

I began writing this book in November 2021, at the peak of our fourth wave of COVID, primarily as a way to boost my own morale, to make me remember why I had devoted my entire medical career to a field of plastic surgery so demanding physically and emotionally. Microsurgery is an independent risk factor for burnout. It is too demanding not to lead to long-term stress. Among microsurgeons there is a high rate of attrition, with fewer and fewer surgeons performing microsurgery as they age. Indeed, within the American Society of Reconstructive Microsurgery (i.e., ASRM), the largest medical group that represents microsurgeons, membership by age is estimated to drop from 38%, 32%, 18%, to 12% respectively from 35–44, 45–54, 55–64, to 65 years and older. In 2022, of the approximate 8000 plastic surgeons who are board certified by the American Board of Plastic Surgeons (ASPS), it is estimated that only about 10% (approximately 854; data provided by ASRM, May 2022) are members of the ASRM. In other words, few plastic surgeons initially devote themselves to microsurgery, and those who do are less willing to devote themselves to this subspeciality as they mature. This is true even though reconstructive microsurgery offers the greatest good to their patients. Hopefully, this book will remind the surgeon what it means to maintain a passion for your profession and will inspire the disillusioned caregiver how fortunate we are to help others. For the layperson, this book is an insight into the tremendous personal energy and commitment made by everyone on the care team of these life-altering surgeries.

Other books have documented the founding and seminal events of microsurgery. Julia K. Terzis MD, PhD has compiled and written an extensive treatise on the history of microsurgery that details the historical landmarks beginning in the 1950s.[1] The innovations by plastic surgeons, especially in the realm of transplant surgery, have been remarkable. Notable examples include the first successful human kidney transplant on identical twins on December 23, 1954, at the Peter Bent Brigham Hospital (later the Brigham and Women's Hospital) performed by Joseph Murray, MD (1919–2012),[2] an American plastic surgeon; and the first full-face human transplant done by plastic surgeons, led by Maria Siemionow, MD, PhD,[3] of the Cleveland Clinic in December 2008. For his pioneering work in organ transplantation, Dr. Murray was honored with the Nobel Prize in Physiology or Medicine in 1990.

Plastic surgery was arguably not a legitimate or recognized specialty within Surgery until the First World War (1914–1918) when it became recognized as a "Branch of War Surgery." This recognition primarily stems from the work of Sir Harold Delf Gillies (1882–1960). The first chapter begins with Sir Gillies in order to introduce basic plastic surgery principles. It then traces the emergence and evolution of microsurgery to put the subsequent chapters, complexity, and advances in perspective.

Microsurgery traces its origins from both Transplant Surgery and Vascular Surgery. It is used in the patient who loses a breast from cancer, the patient whose mandible or tongue is resected to treat an oral cavity cancer, or the patient who needs microvascular reconstruction of his/her extremity or face after a motor vehicle accident, gunshot wound, or animal attack. These patients whose lives have been shattered by cancer and severe trauma hope their lives and bodies will be restored to normal by our surgery. This book tells the stories of these patients, illuminates some general truths about how patients physically and psychologically heal, and demonstrates some of the limitations of reconstruction.

As a medical student, I was fortunate to be schooled in the Yale System of medical education. The core concept of the Yale System is that individuals require guidance and stimulation rather than compulsion or competition to succeed. The corollary of this concept is that students must assume more than the usual responsibility for their education. Memorization of facts was far less important than a well-rounded education in fundamental principles and the acquisition of a scientific habit of mind. There were no grades and no class rank. To foster a lifelong interest in learning and self-education, each student had to write a research thesis to graduate. The thesis was your opportunity to raise a novel question, to determine a methodology to answer the question, and then to arrive at a conclusion that you could defend. My dissertation, "The United Company of Barbers and Surgeons of London, 1540–1745: Union and Disintegration," revolved around the question of how surgeons asserted a legitimate right to be recognized as part of a learned profession, and to be considered not just tradesmen (i.e., barber-surgeons) working with their hands.[4] To understand this question and to understand the historical context of surgical education, in 1989 I enrolled as a graduate student at the University of Cambridge in England to obtain a Master of Philosophy (MPhil) in the History of Medicine. Yale allows and encourages their medical students to take an extra year or two off to pursue additional graduate study.

For many centuries, surgery was isolated as a craft performed by barbers. The university-educated Doctors of Physic (i.e., Doctors of Internal Medicine) would not demean themselves to touch, cut, or clean patients. By advancing their formal education both at university and in established hospital programs and pursuing practical surgical experience in the military, surgeons in England were eventually able to establish themselves as distinct both from their counterparts, the barber-surgeons, as well as from the Doctors of Physic. The perspective gained from my dissertation taught me an important lesson. To be a surgeon, in particular a microsurgeon, you must work like a barber-surgeon, be educated like a Doctor of Physic, and be willing to fail. Microsurgeons actually make things; they get their hands dirty. They build body parts to replace what is missing. The initial chapters of this book will illustrate what can and cannot be done to remake faces, extremities, and breasts to their original, undamaged states. A separate chapter on the reconstruction that is necessary after a gunshot wound will demonstrate the devastating, long-lasting effects of gun violence.

What distinguishes the University of Cambridge from some of America's great universities, such as Harvard and Yale, is the high degree of specialization that students pursue at Cambridge immediately upon enrollment. By focusing on a select field of study, the student can obtain an extraordinary depth of knowledge in their chosen field at a younger age. Moreover, lectures are rather "free-floating". Once you decide on a topic or question to research, you literally decide what relevant lectures and courses that you wish to attend. There are no grades in these courses; rather, it is an opportunity for you to learn what is important for your topic of research. On a weekly basis you meet with your academic advisor or a small group of faculty and students in your academic field to discuss your ideas and to challenge your conclusions. It was your responsibility to determine what was important and how to defend it.

Both Yale and Cambridge taught me what I think has become my greatest strengths as a plastic surgeon. You must assume the ultimate responsibility of your education and how to advance your knowledge. In surgery, this means anticipating every possible surgical option and outcome. Plan for success, but be prepared for failure. Mike White, MD, Professor and member of the Plastic Surgery Faculty at the University of Pittsburgh, would challenge his residents before each case with the question, "tell me six ways this operation could be done, and why you favor what you have chosen". The corollary of this question is that as a treating surgeon, you do not ask a question unless and until you have reached your limits in trying to answer this question for yourself. If you do not know how to do something or can only imagine how it should be done, then you need to prepare yourself, teach yourself every principle of anatomy, physiology, and surgical detail that could possibly be relevant. Moreover, once you have committed to a surgical plan, you need to critically assess the outcome, possibly by publishing your results.

Clinical wisdom is not necessarily the equivalent of clinical experience. William Osler, MD (1849–1919), one of the four founding professors of Johns Hopkins Hospital, astutely noted, "Each case has its lesson – a lesson that may be, but is not always learnt."[5] Chapter 7, entitled "Value, Options, and Cost of Clinical Research", will underscore some of the lessons that clinical surgery and research offer each other. However, these two endeavors can also be in financial conflict. The economics of funding research versus the time devoted to taking care of patients must be considered as any surgeon plans their career.

Most surgeons at a certain midpoint in their career begin to restrict their practice and do only a certain number of limited procedures with predictable outcomes. Multiple factors, including operating room efficiency (i.e., shorter cases), better reimbursement (i.e., dollars paid per minute of operating), improved clinical outcomes (i.e., high-volume versus low-volume surgeons), and a desire for predictability in personal life, have affected this change in practice. For example, a general surgeon may perform only hernias or cholecystectomies; an orthopedic surgeon just knee replacements or shoulder surgery; and a plastic surgeon just breast augmentations and abdominoplasties. The exceptions to this generalization tend to be those surgeons who focus their practice on trauma and cancer. Each trauma patient presents with a unique set of injuries that cannot be neatly scheduled.

The surgical removal of cancers that require complex reconstruction, in particular of the head and neck (i.e., oral and pharyngeal cancer, extensive skin cancers), requires the surgeon not only to be able to surgically solve the problem but also to always be available to treat any complication or recurrence. These principles of self-education, critical assessment of outcomes, and self-challenge have particular relevance in microsurgery.

In the spirit of the Yale System, one must acknowledge that the most significant teachers are the patients on whom we operate. They change our understanding of suffering and what is truly valuable in life. They change how and on what we focus our energy and study. This book is about courage, education, and the limitations of both patients and surgeons. Patients at their time of trauma or diagnosis do not choose to be profiles in courage, but through their suffering, they often become role models for the surgeons. They show them how to be more emotionally prepared, reaffirm how grateful they should be to be in a position to help, and, one must admit, have given surgeons the opportunity to become technically better, to accept the next surgical challenge, to help the next patient.

There are two audiences for this book. First, plastic surgery is so much more than just cosmetic surgery. Any medical professional who has a casual interest in plastic surgery or wellness will see the wonderful miracles that microsurgery can provide to help patients recover from cancer and trauma. The second audience is doctors and patients (or families) who wish to see what is beyond the "routine explanation" for reconstruction that has been or will be recommended. They will likely recognize their own questions, and possible answers, in the stories of the patients presented. Aspiring microvascular surgeons in plastic surgery and/or otolaryngology – head and neck surgery – will be able to reflect on the importance of microsurgery, its limitations, and the required determination.

Every surgical consultation ends with the question: "What would you do if this was your loved one?" The response involves a deep inward examination. First, can you, the surgeon, reliably perform the operation that you are suggesting? These operations are often not found in a textbook. The surgeon designs them based on the available anatomy and the problem. Second, will the pain, anxiety, and any potential complications introduced by the intervention outweigh the suffering now being experienced by the person in front of you? Third, are your priorities for this patient's outcome in alignment with their wishes?

Allen Richard Selzer, MD (1928–2016), general surgeon and author, poetically said: "To do surgery without a sense of awe is to be a dandy – all style no substance. No part of the operation is too lowly, too menial."[6] Microsurgery is all substance, no fluff. I have had the privilege to devote myself to a profession that I love, the honor of being trusted to give advice, and the gratitude for helping others overcome a life-altering event. I hope this book offers some level of inspiration to the general public, patients, and doctors alike.

REFERENCES

1. Terzis JK. *History of Microsurgery – 5 Generations from 1957*. Lulu, 2008.
2. Murray JE. *Surgery of the Soul: Reflections on a Curious Career*. Science History Publications, 2001.
3. Siemionow M. *Face to Face: My Quest to Perform the First Full Face Transplant*. Kaplan Publishing, 2009.
4. Deleyiannis FWB. The United Company of Barbers and Surgeons of London, 1540–1745: union and disintegration. MPhil thesis, University of Cambridge, 1990.
5. Osler W. "Counsels and Ideals". From *The Writings of William Osler*. Houghton Mifflin. Second edition, Oxford University Press, 1929, p. 152.
6. Selzer R. *Letters to a Young Doctor*. Simon & Schuster, 1982, p. 50.

Chapter 1

Microvascular surgery

Why is this so different and special?

It is in the interface of the specialties that progress is made.

– Joseph Murray, MD
Plastic surgeon, transplant surgeon,
and Nobel Prize winner

On a freezing December morning, Chance, a 9-year-old boy, was found unconscious in his backyard with a German shepherd chewing and eating his face and scalp. The paramedics saved his life. Intravenous lines were placed to give blood and fluids to restore blood pressure and a pulse. A breathing tube was placed to control his airway, and the patient was emergently flown by helicopter to Denver.

On arrival, the entire scalp, left forehead, left cheek, ear, and left eyelids were missing. The remaining head and neck were a matted ball of dried blood, hair, macerated tissue, bone, and dog saliva. As an attending surgeon having treated massive avulsions and gunshot wounds to the face for over 20 years, I had seen and treated nearly every imaginable injury in the face. But this injury made me hesitate and seriously ask myself, "Can I repair this, and what can the family, the child, and I really expect once we have finished the reconstruction."

I knew that I must make a plan. I began to survey the body to determine what parts of the legs, arms, back, or abdomen I could detach and transfer to the head and face to reconstruct what remained.

Every surgeon, especially those treating trauma, understands that you do not let fear stop you. However, there is an important caveat in the context of devastating injuries and procedures which you are literally designing de novo. First, you must ask yourself if you are the most qualified and experienced to handle this injury. If not, you are morally obligated to call for assistance and assemble the team most qualified to care for this patient. This is real self-awareness, and one must be honest with oneself and, importantly, be aware of just how good and experienced the surgeons may be that are in your circle of contacts. To paraphrase Stephen Sondheim (1930–2021), American composer, remember also that "nice is different than good". You want an excellent surgeon, not a nice mediocre surgeon. Second, you must define and extrapolate in your own mind how your previous experiences

DOI: 10.1201/9781003538028-2

can aid this patient. You must ask yourself very precisely, "What are steps in this first operation and in the series of operations that you might perform until this patient is healed? What morbidity (i.e., harm) can you potentially cause with each option that you choose?"

Present-day plastic surgery is at its core educated manual labor that can be performed only after years of formal university education followed by additional years of residency and fellowship. Typically, a plastic surgeon will have completed four years of undergraduate education, four years of medical school, and a plastic surgery residency that is 5–7 years long (including internship and possibly 1–2 years of research). Before the early 2000s, the majority of plastic surgeons had also completed a separate residency in another surgical specialty, such as general surgery (5–7 years) or otolaryngology – head and neck surgery (5–7 years), followed by a second residency in plastic surgery (2–3 additional years). Presently, integrated plastic surgery residency programs now offer graduating medical students the opportunity to begin a 5- to 7-year program without the need to complete a separate residency in general surgery or otolaryngology. Fellowships within the subspecialities of plastic surgery, such as pediatric plastic surgery, craniofacial surgery, microsurgery, and hand surgery are an additional 1–2 years. After your formal training, real expertise within your chosen subspeciality of plastic surgery comes only after years and thousands of hours operating and treating patients. Expertise requires enormous time.

The term "plastic surgery" comes from the Greek word *plastikos*, referring to an object that could be shaped or sculpted. Plastic surgery was arguably not a legitimate or recognized specialty within surgery until the First World War (1914–1918), when it became recognized as a "Branch of War Surgery." This recognition stems primarily from the work of Sir Harold Delf Gillies. A New Zealand surgeon, Gillies had studied medicine in England at Gonville and Caius College, University of Cambridge; practiced as an otolaryngologist in London; and was posted to France in 1915 with the Royal Army Medical Corps.[1,2]

During the First World War, heavy artillery and machine guns created injuries of a severity and scale not seen before. Shells filled with shrapnel were meant to maim, to inflict as much damage as possible. Trench warfare resulted in a high number of survivable but devastating facial injuries. Shrapnel would literally tear faces off. "Whenever the head of a careless soldier, possibly with steel helmet tipped back, peeped put of the trench and a ray of moonlight touched his white face, there was another patient for (us)," Gillies wrote (p. 11).[2] Such injuries could not adequately be treated at the front. Wounds were typically pulled together with stitches or bandages to stop the bleeding and then allowed to heal secondarily. Missing tissue, such as skin, muscle, or bone, was not replaced. Wounds healed with horrible contractures that pulled faces into grotesque scars. Soldiers with jaw or cheek wounds were often left with gaping holes with the inability to chew or hold food in their mouths. Patients with nasal injuries were often left with a deep hole in their central face where the nose should have been.

The National Army Museum in Chelsea, London, records the experience of John Glubb, an English soldier, who was hit by a shell fragment in August 1917:

> The floodgates in my neck seemed to burst, and the blood poured out in torrents ... I could feel loosely in my left cheek, as though I had a chicken bone in my mouth. It was, in reality, half my jaw, which had been broken off, teeth and all, and was floating about in my mouth.[3]

On his return to England, Gillies set up a special surgical ward for facial and jaw injuries at the Cambridge Military Hospital in the town of Aldershot (Hampshire, England). In France, with the war still raging, soldiers with facial injuries were tagged with labels that directed their transport and care back to Gillies in England. In 1917, Gillies established the Queen's Hospital in Sidcup, London, as the first hospital dedicated to the treatment of facial injuries. Gillies assembled a multidisciplinary team consisting of dentists, anesthetists, mask makers, and prosthodontists to assist in the care of wounds affecting the teeth, jaws, and face. Artists and photographers were employed to illustrate the before and after of surgical operations. In 1920, he published his seminal work, *Plastic Surgery of the Face Based on Selected Cases of War Injuries of the Face Including Burns*.[1] The book begins with a discussion of the principles of plastic surgery. The first principle, the one which Gillies believed should govern the whole treatment of facial injuries, was that

> normal tissue should be replaced as early as possible, and maintained in its normal position. ... Every effort should be made to replace tissues in their normal position by stiches, strapping, head-gear apparatus, nasal supports and splints, but never into abnormal positions.
>
> (pp. 5–6)

In planning the reconstruction for the patient who arrived from France with his wound sutured or scarred across his face, the first step was to recreate the wound by releasing and resecting the scarred tissue. The reconstruction was then designed from "within, outwards". The lining membrane (i.e., the mucosa of the mouth or the nose) was first replaced by advancing mucosal flaps from intact, uninjured sites or by introducing new skin as skin grafts or flaps to replace the missing epithelium. The next step was to replace or build up the supporting structure of the face. "The replacement should be as nearly as possible in terms of the tissue lost, i.e., bone for bone, cartilage for cartilage, fat for fat, etc." (p. 6). Finally, the surgeon should replace the skin covering. At the time there was little choice in the way of skin reconstruction; one had to choose between a skin graft or a pedicled skin flap.

Prior to Gillies, surgeons had demonstrated an extensive experience with skin grafts. Skin grafts are either partial (containing the more superficial layers of the skin) or full thickness (containing all of the layers of the skin).

Flaps are sections of tissue that contain full thickness skin, the fat below the skin, and possibly the fascia and muscle below. The reliability and success of these flaps are based on capturing and maintaining the blood supply which enters the base of the flap. This base and the blood supply are referred to as the pedicle of the flap. Flaps could be raised next to the wound and swung over to the defect to replace the missing tissue without disconnecting their blood supply in the pedicle. For small defects, such as of the lips, cheeks, or eyelids, Gilles outlined how to design and use these flaps. Results were then illustrated with case series with pre-operative and post-operative photographs.

These flaps were often raised without a known consideration or identification of the blood supply. Wisdom was gained by trying what might be successful. As Gillies acknowledged in the introduction to his book,

> There is hardly an operation – hardly a single flap – in use today that has not been suggested a hundred years ago. But our work is original in that all of it has had to be built up again de novo. ... It has been illuminating to discover the impracticability of many of these, which would appear to have been put forward on the study of one case only, or even on purely theoretical grounds.
>
> (pp. 3–4)

By treating thousands of war injuries, through trial, failure, and success, Gillies determined the operations that worked.

Blood supply was recognized to have a critical importance, and Gillies highlighted that when a known artery was placed in the base of a flap, blood supply was more robust and reliable. For example, in nasal reconstruction, Gillies described the use

> of a long flap containing the anterior branch of the superficial temporal artery, based on the pre-auricular region. ... The blood supply of this flap is remarkable; its nourishing vessel spouts freely when the tubed portion is severed from the new nose.
>
> (p. 19)

However, the vascular anatomy of flaps, especially the finer details of how perfusion is delivered to the skin from the deeper vascular structures, was not yet described.

We know today that there are networks of blood vessels which deliver perfusion to the skin. These networks of blood vessels are spread like spider's webs within the skin and the superficial fat just below the skin. Within the skin, they are too small and too arborized to be detached and then sewn back together, even with the aid of an operating microscope. However, these networks can always be followed deeper and deeper into the body to determine their source. The direct source to the skin is a perforator which

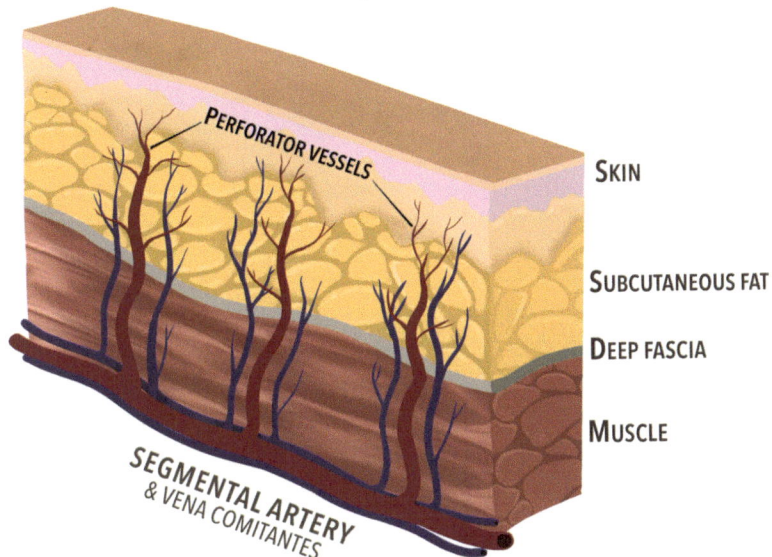

Figure 1.1 Typical anatomy and course of musculocutaneous arteries.

A sizeable segmental (i.e., axial) artery typically runs underneath a muscle and sends perforating branches through the muscle, fascia, and fat to perfuse the skin.

contains an arteriole (i.e., a small artery) and venules (i.e., small veins). These perforators travel through the muscles of the body and within the fascia that wrap and separate the muscles. They then exit the muscle and the deep fascia to perfuse the superficial fat and skin (Figure 1.1). These perforators originate from even larger blood vessels (i.e., an axial/segmental blood supply) which are deeper in the body. Perforators and axial vessels can be seen with the naked eye or with an eye aided with Loupe magnification (i.e., 2x to 3x magnification) and, importantly for microsurgery, can be divided and then reconnected to a different artery and vein in a different part of the body.

The details of these vascular networks were not fully known by Gillies, but the fundamental anatomy had been published nearly 30 years earlier. In 1889, a 23-year-old German medical student at the Kaiser Wilhelm University in Strassburg, Carl Manchot (1866–1932), published his classic work, *Die Hautarterien des Menschlichen Korper* (The Cutaneous Arteries of the Human Body).[4] His scientific methods have been lost, but whatever his technique, Manchot injected a substance, possibly India ink or some form of latex, into the arterial system of his cadaver specimens, which he then dissected. His anatomical drawings illustrated the origin of these skin vessels from the deeper muscles and the surrounding fascia. They showed the cutaneous arteries, their main divisions, and the much deeper vessels

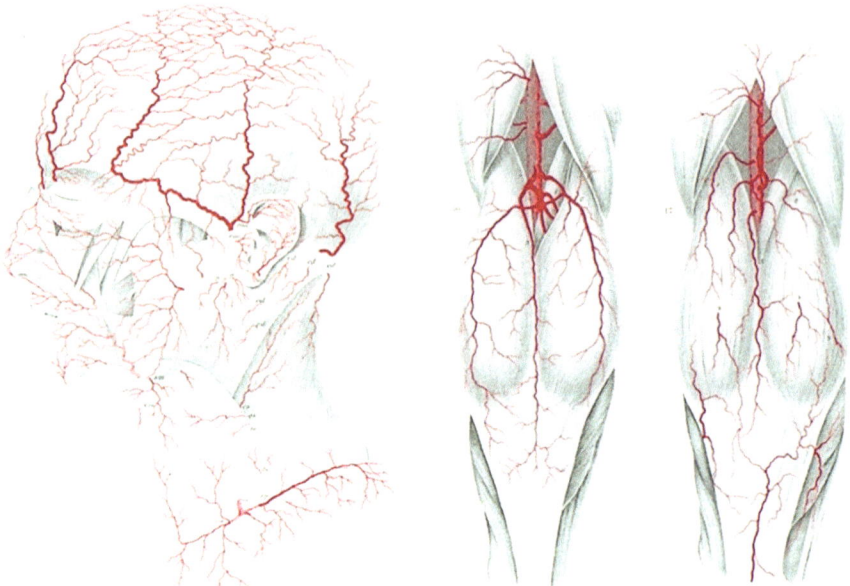

Figure 1.2 Manchot's anatomical sketches: (left) of the head and neck; (right) of the calf.

Originally published in 1889, Manchot's manuscript showed the origin and branching patterns of the cutaneous arteries of the entire body. Remarkedly, the work was completed in 6 months during a funded assistantship from October 1886 to April 1887 at the Anatomy Institute of the Kaiser Wilhelm University. Though awarded the grand prize of the annual medical student competition for research (along with cash award of 300 marks), Manchot's work was largely unknown until the middle of the 20th century. [Reprinted from *The Cutaneous Arteries of the Human Body* (figures 9, 16, and 17; pp. 125 and 131) by Carl Manchot (translated by Jovanka Ristic and William D. Morain), 1983. (Copyright 1983 by Springer Nature]

from which the smaller vessels originated (Figure 1.2). These anatomical details laid the foundation for the revolution in skin flap design which occurred during the next century. However, perhaps because of a lack of communication between surgeons and anatomists, and because he did not speak German, Gillies was not aware of these studies.

If the two had ever met, Manchot likely would have told Gillies that the human skin is not randomly supplied by blood. There is precise mosaic of arterial territories that are supplied by highly predictable arteries. If one wishes to transfer skin or muscle in a flap, these vessels needed to be respected and not divided to ensure the greatest blood supply. The perforating vessels that exit the muscle to supply the overlying fascia, fat, and skin were critical for perfusion.

Manchot's work remained dormant for decades in the English-speaking world. Gillies, like the majority of plastic surgeons of his generation, continued to rely mainly on length-to-width ratios to ensure flap viability. Geometric trial, instead of the anatomical certainty provided by the inclusion of an artery, was the principle for flap design. Experience had shown that flaps with a wide base and short length were more likely to have reliable perfusion at their ends than flaps with narrow bases. It is now known that this is because more of that network of blood vessels below the dermis and facia (i.e., more perforators) are likely to be captured in a wide base versus a narrow base. It was an established plastic surgery principle that the viable length of a skin flap was proportional to the width of the pedicle.

Beginning in the 1960s, Manchot's concept of skin vascular territories was reintroduced and incorporated into the surgical design of skin flaps. During this time, a revolutionary step in this progress was the experimental work done by Stuart Milton (1935–1971), who was investigating flaps for his PhD dissertation in the laboratories of the Nuffield Department of Surgery of the Radcliffe Infirmary in Oxford, England.[5,6] Milton raised skin flaps on the flanks of pigs and then quantitated and examined how much of the flap survived based on their length and width. What was most revolutionary was that Milton anatomically correlated flap survival with vascular anatomy. To his surprise, and contrary to the prevailing plastic surgery wisdom, Milton showed that the surviving length of a skin flap was not directly proportional to its width. Long and narrow skin flaps could safely be raised as long as they were based on a known vessel with the vessel entering the base of the flap. Additionally, he cut the skin at the base of the flap to make the flap an "island" and discovered that these "island" flaps still survived to the same or greater length as long as they contained a segmental artery that passed deep into the skin to enter the midportion of the flap.

According to William D. Morain, MD (author and retired Professor of Plastic Surgery, Dartmouth-Hitchcock Medical Center) who translated Manchot's text into English in 1983, Milton "was fascinated with Manchot and recognized at once the remarkable achievement in the German's book. ... He arranged for Brian Ross, a colleague at Oxford, to do an English translation of Manchot's book from which to work" (p. 51).[4] In his American travels, Milton carried this English translation with him and introduced the work to multiple American plastic surgeons, including Rollin Daniel, who is credited with copublishing the first case of reconstruction using a free skin flap, and Dr. William Grabb, Head of the Section of Plastic Surgery at the University of Michigan (1977–1982) and editor of one of the main plastic surgery textbooks of the time. This dissemination of knowledge of skin vascular anatomy led to an explosion of publications in the 1970s and 1980s describing the vascular anatomy and utility of flaps, pedicled and free, that could be used for reconstruction.

McGregor and Morgan's classification of axial and random pattern skin flaps in the 1970s was one of the first and most important publications, particularly because the research was done in living patients, not cadavers.[7] As described in their landmark 1973 article, 14 patients undergoing surgery for various procedures (i.e., hernia repair, neck dissection, cartilage harvest) were injected with fluorescein into a known, named artery: the internal mammary artery, superficial temporal artery, superficial circumflex artery, or superficial inferior epigastric artery. Fluorescein is a highly fluorescent substance which emits light in the green-yellow range when exposed to ultraviolet (UV) light. Once each artery was cannulated and injected with fluorescein, the authors examined and determined what areas of skin emitted fluorescence. These would be the areas of skin perfused by the axial artery. Typically, "the areas of fluorescence approximated for an ellipse lying along the line of the injected vessels". The authors concluded, and subsequent clinical trials have shown to be true, that flaps that remain within these vascular territories of the axial arterial-venous pedicle should be a "safe flap" (i.e., without flap necrosis).

Advancing Manchot's concept of skin vascular territories, in 1987 Taylor and Palmer introduced the concept of angiosomes which separated the body into 3D blocks of tissue, each fed by a source artery and drained by specific veins.[8,9] Multiple subsequent publications displayed in greater detail the distinct angiosomes in different parts of the body. Taylor and his colleagues devised an injection technique using radio-opaque lead oxide. The common carotid and femoral arteries of fresh cadavers were injected with the lead oxide solution to achieve total body and/or limb perfusion. The infusion was judged to be complete when the mucosal membranes of the oral cavity and the incisions within the pulps of the fingers and toes turned bright orange. The anatomy of the arterial supply to the skin, muscle, and periosteum of the bone was then examined. Using dissections, radiographs, and color coding, Taylor and his colleagues then mapped out the units of tissue (skin, subcutaneous fat, fascia, muscle, and bone) that were perfused by each source artery. Importantly, their work also showed that connections of small arterioles between adjacent angiosomes occur within tissue (i.e., within the skin and muscles), not between them. Because the skin, bone, and most muscles receive perfusion from multiple source arteries (i.e., are within multiple angiosomes), if one artery is interrupted or damaged by disease, trauma, or flap harvest, the circulation to the surrounding tissue can still be reconstituted. The anastomoses between angiosomes act as vital shunts between the major source arteries. Thus, with an understanding of these angiosomes, a flap could reliably be harvested, and importantly, it could be done such that the tissue at the harvest site could heal without creating a wound or lasting injury.

These investigations were meticulous and time consuming. The dissection of just the angiosomes of the lower extremity spanned over 2 years (Figure 1.3). The angiosome concept still serves as the anatomic basis for the design of all flaps, either local or free. The key concept to reliably raising any skin flap is capturing a robust perforator in the flap. Through Ian Taylor's work, surgeons now had well-described maps to assist them in finding this blood supply.

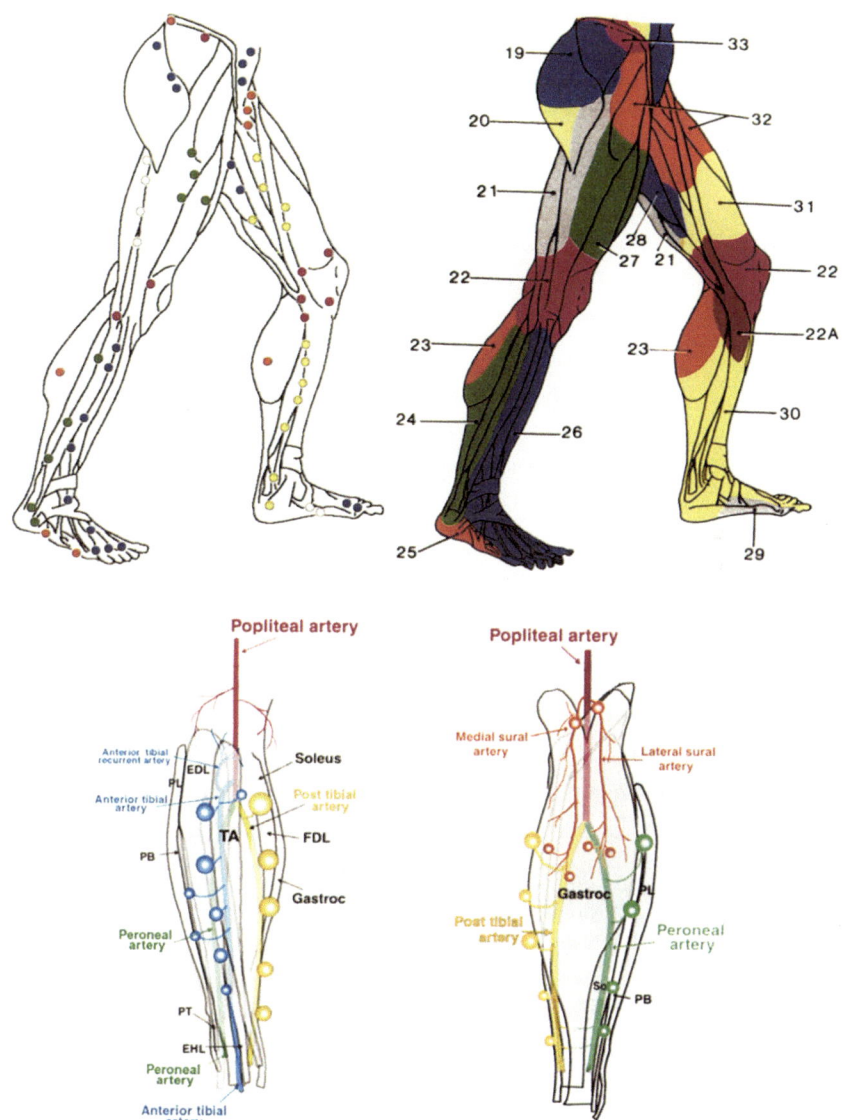

Figure 1.3 The angiosomes and cutaneous perforators of the lower extremity.

The colored spheres are sited at the points of emergence of the cutaneous perforators from the deep fascia and depict the relative size of these vessels. In the upper right figure, the angiosomes of the leg are the popliteal (22), descending genicular (22A), sural (23), peroneal (24), anterior tibial (26), and posterior tibial (30). EDL, extensor digitorum longus; EHL, extensor hallucis longus; FDL, flexor digitorum longus; PB, peroneus brevis; PL, peroneus longus; PT, peroneus tertius; So, soleus; TA, tibialis anterior. [Reprinted from Angiosomes of the leg: anatomic study and clinical implications (Figure 1.4, p.603) by Ian Taylor and Wei Pan. *Plast Reconstr Surg*. 1998. (Copyright 1998 by Wolters Kluwer Health Inc.)]

To Gillies, working 70 years before Ian Taylor's work, what remained a daunting challenge was how to reconstruct defects with large amounts of skin missing. Small flaps rotated from the surrounding zones of the face often could not provide enough skin, or the raising of a skin flap from one site of the face would create a new defect that then needed reconstruction. Through trial and error, Gilles determined which pedicled flaps raised from sites distant from the facial defect, usually from the chest, neck, or scalp, could reliably be used for facial reconstruction. He referred to these as flaps with a "tubed" pedicle because he would sew the edges of the flap together into a tube. The sewing of the edges together helped prevent the undersurface of the flap, the raw area without skin, from bleeding, weeping fluid, and becoming infected. Once the "tubed flap" had healed to the site of the injury and had established a new blood supply from the surrounding tissue, the base of the flap (i.e., the original blood supply) was then divided.

To demonstrate these methods of flap reconstruction, teaching models and wax casts were created. Figure 1.4 demonstrates a 3D printed copy of a wax teaching model from 1917. The original model belongs to the Royal College of Surgeon's Hunterian Museum in London.[3] Many, if not all, of these tubed, pedicled flaps likely captured a perforator in their base. This is why they could successfully survive on a narrow base. However, at the time, their blood supply was poorly understood. They worked, and as a result, for decades "tubed flaps" were a primary means of reconstruction.

What has changed remarkably is our present ability to completely divide a blood supply (i.e., to divide the pedicle) and to reattach the vessels. Thus, flaps no longer have to be tubed, done in multiple stages, and limited to tissue that is relatively near the defect. Because the arteries and the veins that provide the blood supply to a flap are so small (usually 1–3 mm), an operating microscope is routinely used to perform the anastomosis (i.e., the reattachment). These operations are referred to as microvascular surgery.

The origins of microvascular surgery (i.e., the sewing of small blood vessels under a microscope) can be traced to fundamental surgical techniques developed for suturing blood vessels in the late nineteenth and early twentieth centuries. In 1894, the president of France, Sadi Carnot, was assassinated in Lyon. Carnot was stabbed in the abdomen and bled to death from a laceration of the portal vein. The prevailing surgical wisdom at that time was that Carnot could not have been saved because the repair of such a vascular injury was not possible. Alexis Carrel, a medical student at the University of Lyon at that time, speculated that this vascular injury could indeed be treated if we could determine how best to repair blood vessels. Inspired by sewing lessons that he took from an embroideress, he then proceeded to develop the extremely fine needles and threads that could be used for repair. He published his first article of vascular anastomoses and methods in 1902,[10] including the technique of "triangulation", using three stay sutures as traction points to minimize damage to the vascular wall, while

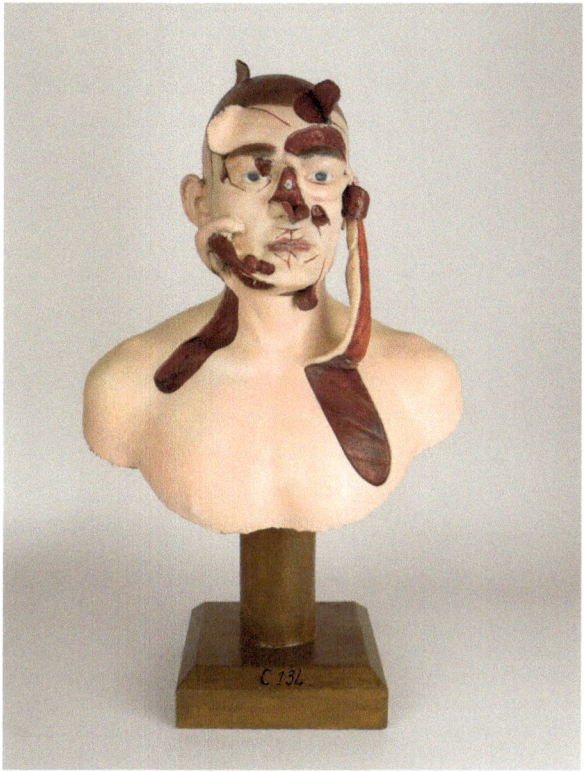

Figure 1.4 Facsimile of a 1917 wax teaching model of "tubed flaps" for facial reconstruction.

This teaching model was made by Sergeant Thomas H Kelsey for the New Zealand Medical Corps facial and jaw injury unit, 1917. It shows how to design "tubed flaps" from the chest, neck, forehead, and scalp. In the first stage of reconstruction the "tubed flap" would be transferred to the face to replace the missing tissue. The next stage of reconstruction would typically involve dividing the base of the flap and leaving the distal end of the flap as replacement for the missing facial tissue. (Image Courtesy of the National Army Museum, London)

suturing blood vessels (Figure 1.5). These techniques are still widely used today in vascular surgery and were responsible for Carrel's receiving the Nobel Prize in 1912.[11,12]

Carrel also published in 1905 what could be described as the first experimental free flap.[13] He transplanted a dog's kidney by dividing the renal vessels, removing the kidney from the abdomen, and then sewing the kidney into the neck by reattaching the renal artery to the carotid artery and the renal vein to the external jugular vein. The ureter was implanted into a small opening in the skin above the sternum. Carrel then described how blood flow was restored to the kidney and urine was then produced. In his 1905 paper, Carrel labeled the

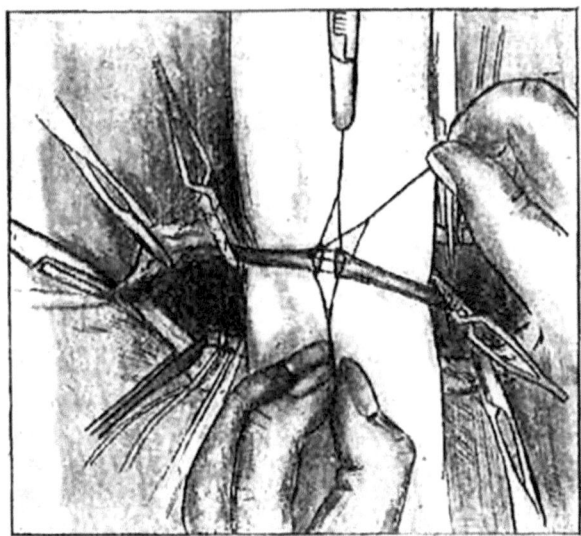

Figure 1.5 Triangulation method of vascular end-to-end anastomosis by Dr. Carrel.
Three stay sutures are placed 120 degrees from each other around the circumference of the vessels. Gentle traction on 2 of the sutures at a time allows evenly spaced and everting sutures to be placed. Sewing of the vessels was done without the aid of operating microscope and limited usually to vessels greater that 7mm in diameter. [Reprinted from *Blood-vessel Surgery and its Application* (figure 29, p.45) by Charles Claude Guthrie CC, 1912. (Public Domain)]

transfer of organs within the same animal as auto-transplantation and characterized the factors that affect a successful auto-transplant.

> The life of the transplanted organs depends almost entirely on the circulation. If the vessels become obliterated, gangrene destroys the organ. Obliteration can occur very easily. It may be produced by a great many causes; for instance, injury to the endothelium by the forceps, the needles or the clamps of temporary hemostasis, clots on the perforating stitches, fall of the external sheath in the opening of the vessel, and above all, lack of perfect asepsis.[13]

This auto-transplantation of an organ or body part within the same animal (i.e., patient) is in its essence what microvascular surgeons do today. It is called free tissue transfer, because the tissue and its blood supply are completely detached (i.e., made "free") and then reattached. It is transplant surgery within the same patient. The introduction of the operating microscope in the 1920s, subsequent microscope innovations such as coaxial illumination, higher magnification, and a motorized zoom, and finer surgical instruments and suture have made these transfers reliable. With each new innovation, it became more obvious that the successful anastomoses of smaller and smaller vessels were possible.

In 1960, Julius Jacobsen, MD, then at the University of Vermont, is credited with introducing the use of the operating microscope for small vessel surgery and is often acknowledged as the Father of Microsurgery.[14–18] Working on a study on canines that required dividing the carotid artery, Jacobsen initially could not achieve consistent success in anastomosing the divided ends. At the time it was commonly thought that arteries smaller than 7 mm in diameter could not be anastomosed reliably. However, after borrowing an operating microscope from ENT surgery, Jacobsen soon realized that magnification, rather than manual dexterity, was the primary limiting factor. His patency rates eventually reached 100% with vessels averaging between 1.4 mm and 3.2 mm in diameter in rabbit and canine models.

In an interview recorded by the Society for Vascular Surgery in 2011, Jacobsen recounted the "aha" moment that led to his realization of the utility of using a microscope for small vessel vascular surgery.[19] Having applied to 23 medical schools and having been rejected by all 23, Jacobsen proceeded to do a year of research studying paramecia, unicellular organisms found in ponds, with a leading cell physiologist, Dr. L.V. Heilbrunn, at the University of Pennsylvania. "Bent over a microscope all day, I did some research on paramecia, which excited the department. As a result, when I reapplied to medical school. … This time I was accepted to every place I applied." The use of a microscope became second nature. In analyzing the reason for the traditional teaching that arteries smaller than 7 mm in diameter could not be successfully anastomosed, Jacobsen summarized, "the eye could not see to tell the hand what to do or, to put it another way, a small error in an aortic anastomosis was of no significance but the same error in a small artery would account for failure."

With this insight, and in conjunction with the Karl Zeiss company which was the maker of the eye/ear microscope, Jacobsen developed the first double binocular microscope in 1961 and named it the "diploscope". In West Germany, the first prototype diploscope was manufactured and then shipped to Vermont. It had a 5- to 40-power magnification capability with a 16-inch working distance that allowed the surgeon and first assistant to work together in the same field without difficulty. About 20 years ago, the original diploscope was donated to the Smithsonian Institution in Washington, D.C.

As Jacobsen continued to work with increasing magnification, he proceeded to develop and advance the technical principles and instruments used for microvascular surgery. The first principle was that fine finger control, not wrist motion, was necessary for precision. Needle holders and scissors were miniaturized and made without the classic ring handles in favor of points of finger control. Initially, some of the instruments were purchased from jeweler supply houses that carried "suitable instruments such as forceps and scissors at a small fraction of the cost of the surgical instrument makers."

To meet the need of suture and needle miniaturization, Ethicon, a surgical suture company, developed a needle that was 5/1000 of an inch in diameter and found a machinist capable of drilling a 1/1000-inch hole into the end of the needle so that a suture of 1/1000-inch diameter could be attached into the base of the needle.

With his diploscope and the newly designed surgical instruments and suture, Jacobsen subsequently proceeded to introduce these microsurgical techniques into the fields of neurosurgery, peripheral vascular surgery, and coronary artery surgery. Within the first year of their introduction, Jacobson and his colleagues had published 18 papers detailing the applications of microvascular surgery.

Remarkably, the first clinical transfer of "free tissue" in a human was done in 1957 without the aid of an operating microscope.[20] Working in the 1950s with canines, the Head and Neck Surgical Oncology Group at Montefiore Hospital in New York City had experimentally designed how to replace the cervical esophagus with a piece of free jejunum (i.e., part of the small intestine). The jejunum would be divided from its blood supply in the abdomen and then transferred to the neck to replace the esophagus. Revascularization was possible by sewing vessels in the neck to the detached vessels of the jejunum. The operation was designed to treat patients with cancer of the esophagus who might undergo surgical resection of their cervical esophagus.

On July 30, 1957, after perfecting the technique in dogs, the procedure was carried out on a 63-year-old man with recurrent squamous cell carcinoma of the cervical esophagus. The mesenteric artery of the jejunum was anastomosed to the left inferior thyroid artery (diameter: 3 mm), and the mesenteric vein was anastomosed to the left common facial vein (Figure 1.6). Unfortunately, the patient sustained a cerebral vascular accident and died on the seventh day after surgery. According to the authors, "At autopsy, the revascularized jejunal segment was pink and viable. ... The jejunal segment was perfused with Diodrast [i.e., a contrast agent] through the inferior thyroid artery, and an x-ray showed patency of its entire vasculature" (Seidenberg, p. 169). Two years later, in 1961, Roberts and Douglass reported on two additional cases of "free jejunal autografts" in the *New England Journal of Medicine*.[21]

The first successful auto-transplantation in man using microvascular techniques was reported in 1972 by McLean and Buncke.[22] At the Naval Hospital in Oakland, California, a 29-year-old man underwent resection of a tumor of his temporal-parietal scalp, leaving a 6- by 8-inch defect which included the outer cortex of the skull. In the report, the authors noted that they previously had carried out with success several experimental procedures on dogs where they had transferred the omentum to the scalp and covered the revascularized omentum with skin grafts. The omentum is an intra-abdominal, large apron-like fold of visceral peritoneum (i.e., a thin lining of tissue attached to the stomach that contains blood vessels,

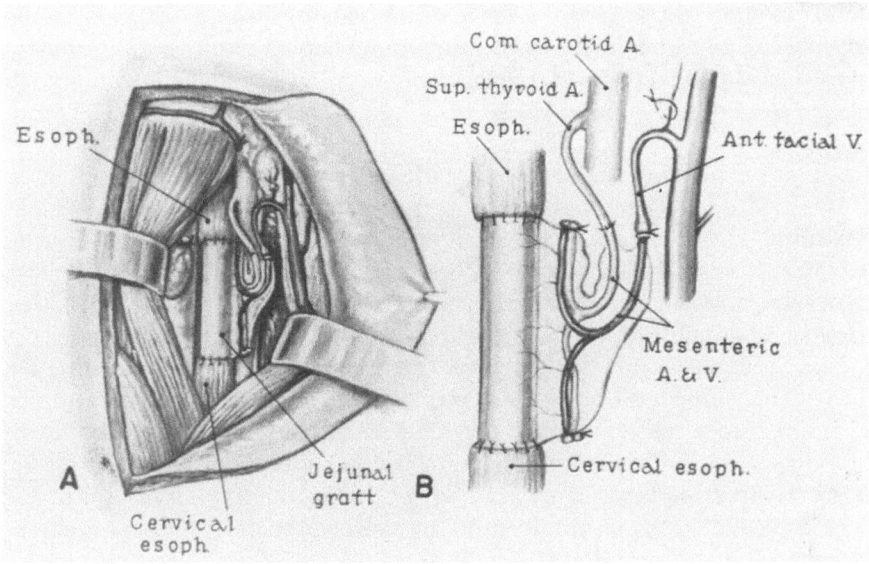

Figure 1.6 Diagram of the first clinical auto-transplant (free flap) in a man, 1957.

A. The resected esophagus has been replaced by a piece of jejunum. B. A more detailed diagram demonstrating the revascularization of the jejunum by reconnecting the blood vessels of the jejunum to blood vessels in the neck. [Reprinted from Immediate reconstruction of the cervical esophagus by a revascularized isolated jejunal segment (Figure 7a, p. 162) by Bernard Seidenberg, Stephen Rosenak, Elliott Hurwitt, et al. *Ann Surg.* 1959 (Copyright 1959 by Wolters Kluwer Health, Inc.)].

lymphatics, and fat). In this first clinical case, the venous and arterial anastomoses were done with the aid of the diploscope, the operating microscope developed by Jacobsen.

Prior to using the omentum for scalp reconstruction, McLean and Buncke commented in their 1972 case report (p. 271):

> we searched elsewhere in the body for a composite tissue transplant having a discrete end-arterial type of vascular supply. The ideal donor sites would be skin and subcutaneous tissue on a single vascular pedicle, the sacrifice of which would be neither disabling nor disfiguring. Such a combination has not been found.

Within the next 2 years, "such combinations", mainly skin free flaps from the lower abdomen, were found and published in multiple reports.

The term "free flap" was coined in 1973 with Ian Taylor and Rollin Daniel's article, "The Free Flap: Composite Tissue Transfer by Vascular Anastomosis".[23,24] In this first successful auto-transplant of a free skin flap in a human, they harvested a flap from the lower abdomen to reconstruct a defect of the right ankle in a 21-year-old male on January 20, 1973. The superficial epigastric vessels of the abdominal flap were successfully anastomosed to the posterior tibial artery and veins in the lower extremity. To plastic surgeons, this provided an exciting alternative to traditional reconstruction. During the next few years, additional clinical cases and a series of free tissue transfer of muscle, bone, and skin were increasingly reported.

By the late 1980s, multiple "routine free flaps" were being used for reconstruction. These mainly included the fibular free flap (first introduced in 1975), the latissimus free flap (1979), the rectus abdominis free flap (1980), the radial forearm free flap (1981), and the parascapular flap (1982). The number of possible donor sites and free flaps continued to expand over the following 30–40 years with dozens of options available to the surgeon. Today, encyclopedias of flaps have been published detailing the indications, anatomy, and surgical techniques.[25,26] Supermicrosurgery (i.e., the sewing of blood vessels less than 0.8 mm in diameter) is presently on the leading edge of reconstructive plastic surgery, offering options to harvest free flaps in less time and with less morbidity and to treat difficult problems, such as lymphedema.

By the end of the 20th century, microsurgery had emerged as a mature surgical specialty. Nearly any body part or piece of tissue that has a distinct blood supply can now be harvested and transferred as a free flap (Figures 1.7 and 1.8). The choice of which free flap to use depends on the type of tissue missing, where in the body the tissue is missing or damaged, and what tissue can reliably and safely be harvested in a particular patient.

In 1888, Sir William Osler became the first Professor of Medicine at the newly founded Johns Hopkins University Medical School in Baltimore.

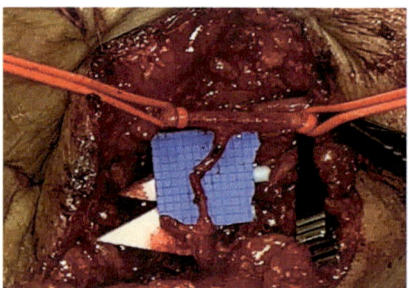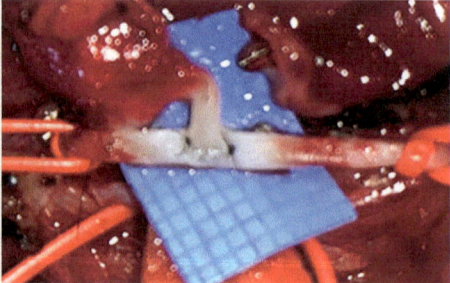

Figure 1.7 Present-day microvascular surgery.

Vessels being anastomosed are typically 1mm - 3 mm in diameter. Each blue square on the background in the picture measures 1mm x 1mm. Left – The medial sural artery from a medial sural artery perforator free flap is about to be sewn end to end into side branch of the posterior tibial artery to reconstruct a defect of the heal. Right – the artery to a gracilis free flap has been sewn end-to-side into the posterior tibial artery to reconstruct a defect around the ankle.

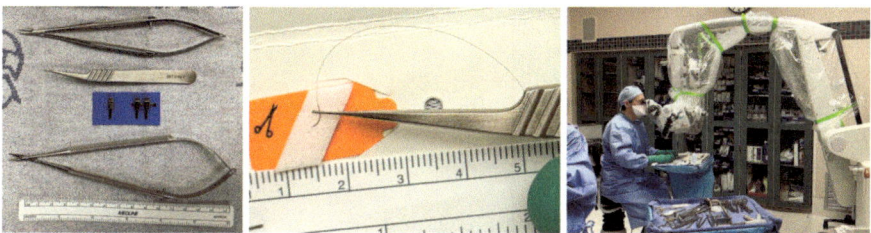

Figure 1.8 Typical microvascular instruments.
Left – needle holder, vessel dilator, microvascular clamps, and scissors. Center- 8.0 Microsuture. Right – Operating microscope.

Generations of physicians have been inspired by his aphorisms, especially those that place a focus on the patient, not the disease. He wrote,

> Medicine is learned by the bedside and not in the classroom. Let not your conceptions of disease come from the words heard in the lecture room or read from the book. See and then reason and compare and control. But see first.[27]

In the following chapters, you will see how surgeons and patients confront life-altering events that only microsurgery can solve. Every operation is a unique challenge learned at the bedside.

REFERENCES

1. Gillies HD. *Plastic Surgery of the Face Based on Selected Cases of War Injuries of the Face Including Burns*. Henry Frowde, Holder and Stoughton, Oxford University Press, 1920.
2. Gillies HD and DR Millard *The Principles and Art of Plastic Surgery*. Little, Brown and Company, 1957.
3. https://www.nam.ac.uk/the-birth-of-plastic-surgery
4. Manchot C. *The Cutaneous Arteries of the Human Body*. Translated by Jovanka Ristic and William D. Morain. Editor: Marie Low. Springer Science and Business Media, LLC, 1983.
5. Milton SH. Pedicled skin-flaps: the fallacy of the length: width ratio. *Br J Surg*. 1970 Jul;57(7):502–508.
6. Milton SH. Experimental studies on island flaps. 1. The surviving length. *Plast Reconstr Surg*. 1971 Dec;48(6):574–578.
7. McGregor IA, Morgan G. Axial and random pattern flaps. *Br J Plast Surg*. 1973 Jul;26(3):202–213.
8. Taylor GI, Palmer JH. The vascular territories (angiosomes) of the body: experimental study and clinical applications. *Br J Plast Surg*. 1987 Mar; 40(2):113–141.

9. Taylor GI, Pan WR. Angiosomes of the leg: anatomic study and clinical implications. *Plast Reconstr Surg.* 1998 Sep;102(3):599–616.

10. Carrel A. technique operatoire des anastomoses vasculaires et la transplantation des visceres. *Lyon Med.* 1902;98:859–864.

11. Sade MD. Transplantation at 100 years: Alexis Carrel, pioneer surgeon. *Ann Thorac Surg* 2005;80:2415–2418.

12. Guthrie CC. *Blood-Vessel Surgery and Its Applications.* Longmans, Green & Co; 1912. Reprinted: Guthrie CC. *Blood-Vessel Surgery and Its Applications.* Legare Street Press, Oct.27, 2022.

13. Carrel A. The transplantation of organ: a preliminary communication. 1905. *Yale J Biol Med.* 2001 Jul–Aug;74(4):239–241.

14. Jacobson JH. Founder's lecture in plastic surgery. *Ann Plast Surg* 2006; 56:471–474.

15. Jacobson JH, Suarez EL. Microsurgery in anastomosis of small vessels. *Surg Forum.* 1960;9:243–245.

16. Jacobson JH, Miller DB, Suarez E. Microvascular surgery: a new horizon in coronary artery surgery. *Circulation.* 1960;22:767.

17. Jacobson JH, Wallman LJ, Schumacher GA, et al. Microsurgery as an aid to middle cerebral artery endarterectomy. *J Neurosurg.* 1962;19:108–115.

18. Yasargil MG, Krayenbuhl HA, Jacobson JH. Microneurosurgical arterial reconstruction. *Surgery.* 1970;67:221–233.

19. www.youtube.com/ Dr Julius H Jacobson II (Interviewed November 18, 2011).

20. Seidenberg B, Rosenak SS, Hurwitt ES, et al. Immediate reconstruction of the cervical esophagus by a revascularized isolated jejunal segment. *Ann Surg.* 1959;149:162–171.

21. Roberts RE, Douglass FM. Replacement of the cervical esophagus and hypopharynx by a revascularized free jejunal autograft. Report of a case successfully treated. *N Engl J Med.* 1961;264:342–344.

22. McLean DH, Buncke HJ Jr. Autotransplant of omentum to a large scalp defect, with microsurgical revascularization. *Plast Reconstr Surg.* 1972;49:268–274.

23. Taylor GI, Daniel RK. The free flap: composite tissue transfer by vascular anastomosis. *Aust N Z J Surg.* 1973 Jul;43(1):1–3.

24. Daniel RK, Taylor GI. Distant transfer of an island flap by microvascular anastomoses. A clinical technique. *Plast Reconstr Surg.* 1973;52:111–116.

25. Deleyiannis FWB. Chapter 162: Microvascular reconstruction of the head and neck. In *Operative Otolaryngology Head and Neck Surgery.* 3rd edition. Eds: Myers EN, Synderman CH. Elsevier Ltd, 2018, pp. 1125–1133.

26. Chase RA. Introduction: The history of vascularized composite-tissue transfers. In *Grabb's Encyclopedia of Flaps*, 4th edition. Eds: Strauch D, Vasconez LO, Herman CK, Lee BT. Wolters Kluwer, 2016, pp. xliii–xlviii.

27. Thayer WS. Osler the teacher. In *Johns Hopkins Hospital Bulletin* 1919: v. 30, p. 198.

Chapter 2

Facial reconstruction

Preserving your sense of self

Of the 11,000 cases that went through Sidcup after August, 1917, and all of those before at Aldershot, there were many in which our results fell far short of the ideal. We noticed that if we made a poor repair for a wretched fellow the man's character was inclined to change for the worse. He would be morose, break rules and give trouble generally. Conversely, if we made good repair, the patient usually became a happy convalescent and soon regained his old character and habits. This seems but to emphasize again the powerful influence that our physical appearance wields over our character. ... Can our general surgeons and our doctor friends realize the ever frightening responsibility of that plan and the irrevocable first cut?[1]

– Sir Harold Delf Gillies OBE, FRCS, 1882-1960
New Zealand otolaryngologist, widely considered the founder of modern plastic surgery

Back to a nearly impossible challenge.

The initial decisions of a plastic surgeon are based on touch and sight, determining whether tissue will live or die, and then deciding when it is safe and optimal to begin the reconstruction. Dead tissue is unmistakable; it is black and does not bleed. Tissue that is white, that bleeds when rubbed, might survive. It has some blood supply. Pink tissue that bleeds freely will live. Infection, hypotension (i.e., low blood pressure), and even the inflammatory response initiated by the trauma can choke this blood supply, leading to further tissue loss. This gradual declaration of survival can take days. The surgeon first decides how much tissue to debride, to cut away with a knife and scissors. Hair, bone, bits of muscle and skin that are free floating, are scrubbed out of the wound with antiseptic. The cutting of necrotic tissue stops when bleeding can clearly be seen in the tissue that still remains.

Chance's left eyelids, lateral left forehead, and brow were black. The left cheek, ear, and the majority of the scalp were missing. A finger inserted into the mouth exited through the wound and appeared where the ear should be.[2]

In an infant, the head and neck are approximately 20% of the total surface of the body. This percentage decreases as the child grows until

DOI: 10.1201/9781003538028-3

adulthood where the head and neck constitute approximately 9% of the total surface area. These percentages are extremely useful for calculating the severity of the injury, as well as for calculating the volume of fluids needed for acute resuscitation. Chance, a 9-year-old boy, had lost approximately 40% of the skin covering his head, face, and neck, approximately 7% of his entire body surface area. Without a cheek, he could not hold food in his mouth. Without eyelids, he could not protect his left eye. His skull was completely exposed like a cadaver's (Figure 2.1).

When I visited with the parents in the intensive care unit (ICU), I would sit on the small couch that was next to the window that also served as a bed for the parents. An oft-repeated counsel is that a doctor should never allow his patient to lose hope. A doctor has the power to offer hope, but with life-threatening issues having prognoses that are somewhat uncertain, one also grapples with the twin issues of truthfulness and optimism. A treating surgeon has the obligation to be sure that no hope that he offers is baseless and that he can deliver the surgical outcome with confidence. One must also articulate the limitations of surgery, the risks, and the eventual outcomes that can realistically be achieved. To tell a parent that their child will never be the same, will never smile on one side of their face, will never have an ear, and will have scar and reconstructed tissue that will forever be seen by the outside world is heartbreaking.

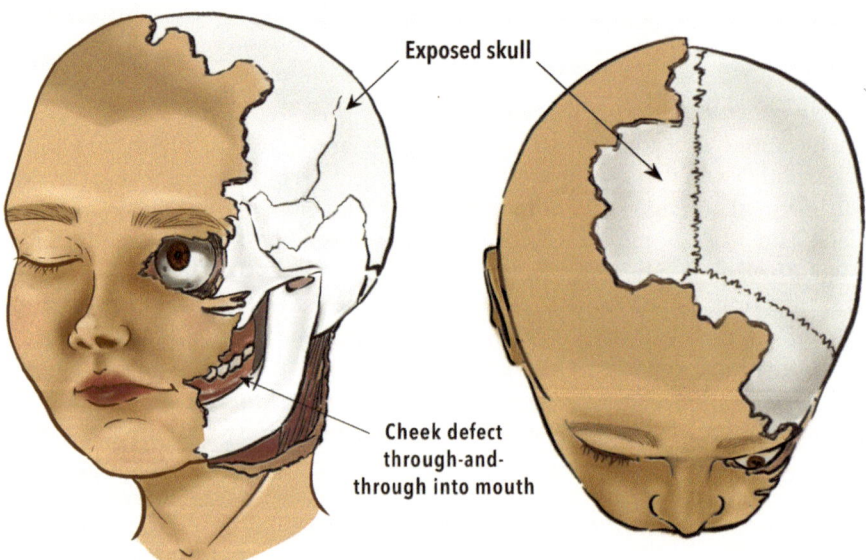

Figure 2.1 Chance's face and skull with defect caused by dog mauling.
The left cheek, ear, and scalp have been bitten and ripped off.

"Chance will be okay. He comes from a loving family and a community that will take care of him." This, one of the first comments from the family, offered a calmness that permeated the next 3 months of treatment. I began to outline the next several operations that I envisioned. I would first take a section of the thigh to fill the hole in the cheek and to seal the mouth from spilling saliva into the face. Then we would proceed with multiple additional free flaps from the back, the other thigh, and abdomen to reconstruct the scalp and forehead (Figure 2.2). The planning of each subsequent operation depended on the success of the previous. Their hope for a successful outcome rested in my ability to do a series of operations that had never been done before.

Every week I raise a multitude of flaps to reconstruct patients who are missing various body parts, and broadly speaking, I know what I will find. Arteries and veins will be where they should be. Skin, fat, and muscle will have a thickness and volume that can be evaluated by touch and observation. Chance was a small, slender child. As I spoke to his parents, I gently pinched his thighs to evaluate the thickness of the skin and fat on top of his thigh muscles. This thickness would match well the thickness of the cheek that was missing. There are, of course, differences (a scar from a previous surgery in one patient, obesity in another), but from mentally cataloguing hundreds of patients for whom a similar flap may have been needed, one creates a profile, a statistical estimate, of how suitable your flap choice is for your present patient.

For Chance, I created his profile and took a deep breath. On the seventh day after the dog attack, we began the first major reconstructive operation.

Optimal facial reconstruction depends on replacing the missing tissue with tissue that is similar in appearance (i.e., color, thickness) and function. There are about 20 paired muscles in the face which are innervated by the seventh cranial nerve, the facial nerve. The facial nerve exits the skull and splits into five primary branches, which then go to the individual muscles of the face to allow the face to smile, frown, and twist into a variety of expressions. Isolated facial nerve injuries can be repaired with direct suturing of the nerves back together or bridged with nerve grafts. For a child born without the ability to smile or for a patient with facial paralysis due to a tumor, a smile gesture can often be restored by transferring a free muscle flap to the face. This free muscle flap can then be re-innervated by connecting a nerve in the face to the nerve of the muscle flap. Contraction of the muscle flap can then simulate the contraction of a normal smile. Routinely, the gracilis muscle is transferred from the thigh, and its nerve, the obturator nerve, is reattached to the facial nerve or to a local motor nerve from a different cranial nerve. Blood supply is reconnected by sewing the pedicle of the gracilis muscle to branches of the carotid artery and jugular vein (Figure 2.3).

Chance was missing his facial musculature and facial nerve, but more acutely, he had direct communication from his mouth to his neck and face. There are literally billions of bacteria in your mouth, with over 700 different

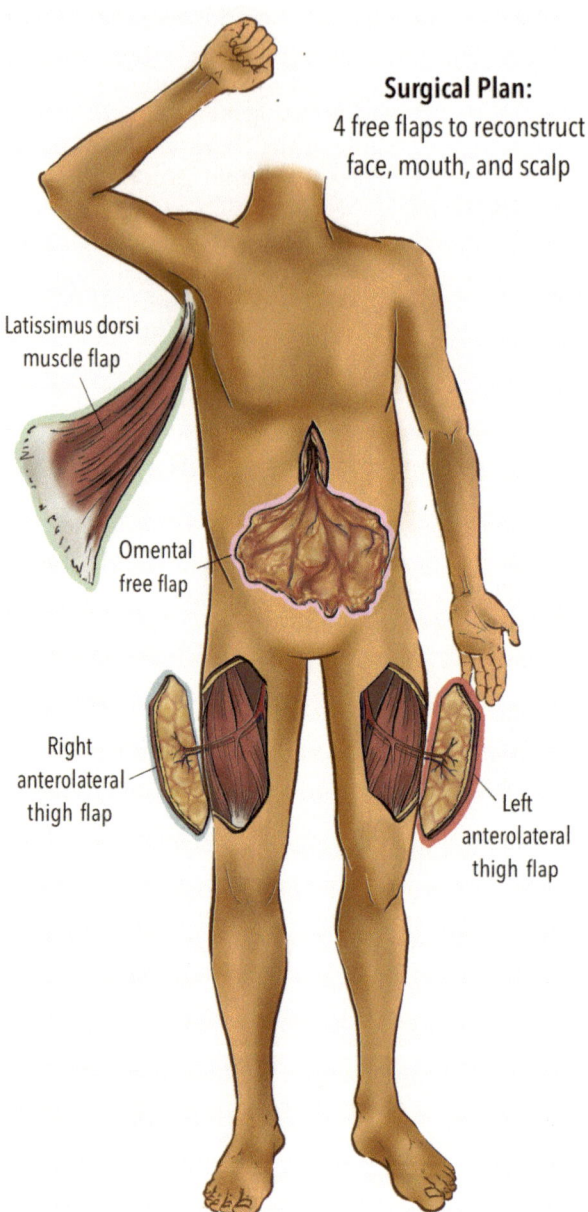

Figure 2.2 Microsurgical plan for reconstruction of the face and scalp.

Facial and scalp reconstruction will be done with 4 free flaps from the legs, abdomen, and back.

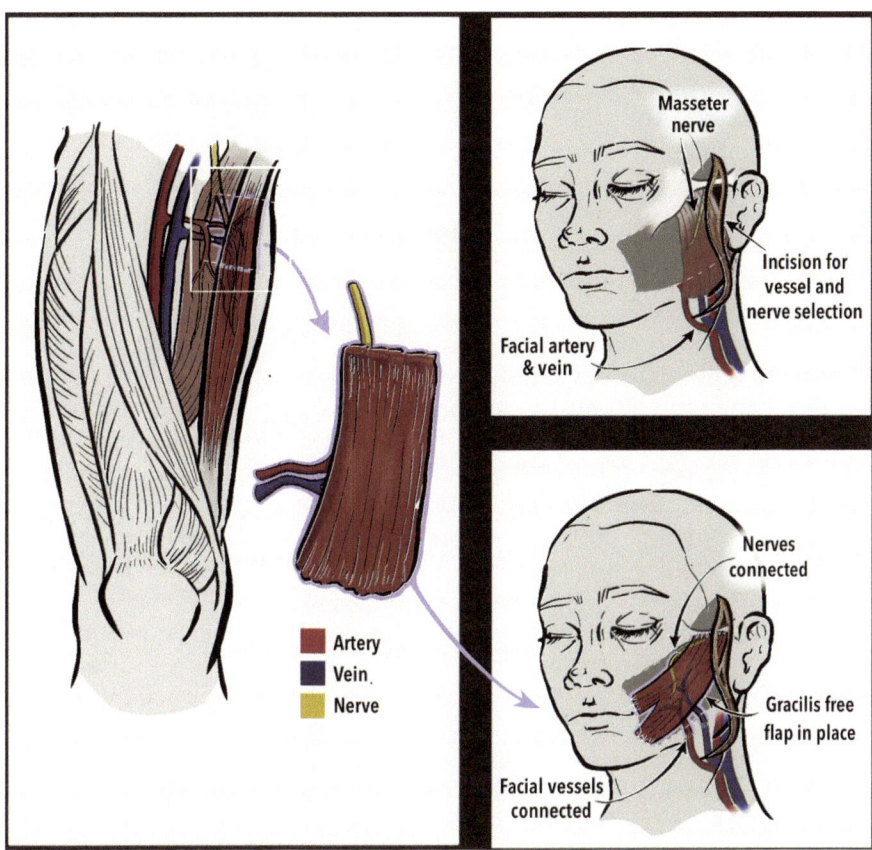

Figure 2.3 Typical facial re-animation surgery with an innervated gracilis free flap.

A patient with a facial paralysis will present with drooping of the involved face. In this example the patient is not missing tissue (i.e., skin and muscle). Treatment can involve placing a gracilis muscle from the thigh (Left Panel) into the face and reattaching the blood vessels and providing a nerve supply from an undamaged nerve (i.e., masseter nerve in this case; Right Panels). This can restore a smile.

types of bacteria. Normally, saliva helps wash away the bacteria and has its own enzymes and antibodies that attack and kill bacteria. Without the ability to swallow and keep saliva in his mouth, the bacteria and saliva puddled in Chance's neck and wound. Infection and continued tissue necrosis are the outcomes unless these are urgently controlled. Facial movement becomes a secondary priority.

Every operation in microvascular surgery is, first, a lesson in geometry. Length, width, and depth of the wound or defect are measured. The location of the recipient vessel for the microvascular anastomosis are estimated.

Will the flap be folded on itself to give two surfaces of skin? How does this folding affect the position of the blood vessels and the resultant contour of the reconstruction? Will the pedicle of the flap be long enough to reach the recipient vessels in the neck? Will vein grafts be needed to reach the recipient vessels? What flap from what part of the body can be thin enough or thick enough to best match the defect? Can the dimensions of the defect be reliably reconstructed with only one flap? If not, what are the second, third, and fourth flap options?

To reconstruct the through-and-through cheek defect, Chance needed a skin paddle the size of a small pancake to resurface the lining of the mouth (i.e., oral cavity buccal mucosa), and a second skin paddle the size of a larger pancake to replace the missing skin from the corner of the mouth to the site of the missing ear. The chosen flap for the oral cavity and cheek reconstruction would be sewn into branches of the carotid and jugular veins in the neck. However, once this first flap had been sewn into position, it would be difficult to again dissect out the vessels in the left neck for any additional microsurgery without putting the anastomosis for the first flap in jeopardy. Thus, if a second flap was needed, it had to be done at the same time as the first to decrease the risk of a complication.

To repair Chance's through-and-through cheek defect, the two stacked pancakes collectively measured 8 cm by 19 cm. For such a large surface area requiring skin, there is primarily one free skin flap that can reliably reconstruct this defect without being too thick and difficult to fold. This is the anterolateral thigh free (ALT) skin flap based on skin perforators from the descending branch of the lateral circumflex artery and veins, which are blood vessels that exit from the profundus artery and vein deep in the thigh.

Most of us have heard the expression "measure twice, cut once". In plastic surgery, this idiom is a practical warning with real consequences if not followed to the extreme. It means measuring the defect anticipating the change in size and shape created by movement (i.e., mouth opening, chewing), wound scarring, and the need to be sure your pedicle is covered by healthy vascularized tissue. Previous experience had driven this message home.

Back in 2006, I was consulted to care for an elderly patient who presented with large buccal oral mucosal cancer eroding through the skin of the cheek. To reconstruct the through-and-through cheek defect that resulted from the resection of the tumor, I designed a radial forearm free flap (RFFF) from the arm to reconstruct the cheek. With the patient asleep under anesthesia and the mouth partially opened, the flap was removed from the arm and inset into the defect on the face. The vessels from the RFFF were tunneled underneath the skin to the neck, and the microscope was brought into the room. The radial artery was then sewn to the facial artery, and the cephalic vein (i.e., the primary superficial vein draining the RFFF) was sewn into the internal jugular vein. With the anastomoses done, the microvascular clamps were released. Instantly, the flap turned pink with healthy bleeding on the skin paddles. The patient went to the intensive care unit, and I was thrilled to tell the family that the operation was a success.

But what a miscalculation! This success was short-lived. As the patient awoke from general anesthesia and sedation, he began to smile, grimace, and open his mouth to talk and eat. The flap was too small. With each gesture, the suture line began to stretch and was put under tension. On the seventh day after surgery, the suture line most lateral on the cheek separated. I could place my pinky finger through the separation into the mouth. With restricting the patient's diet and initiating wound care, the fistula into the mouth gradually shrunk over the next 4 weeks until it reached the width of a pencil. Once the patient resumed an oral diet, small amounts of saliva continued to exit the patient's cheek. The patient decided that he did not want any more surgery. He was left with the hole that I had created.

I brought the memory of this case with me to the operating room as I designed the flap to reconstruct Chance's cheek. In the operating room, a template was drawn on a surgical towel which outlined the dimension and positions of the defects in the mouth and skin. The sizes of the defects were measured with Chance's cheek and lips placed on maximum stretch as if doing a wide yawn. This template was then cut into the shape and size of the combined defect. The flap was designed to be folded on itself so the skin could be placed in the mouth and then draped into the cheek. This folding also required that extra skin be harvested to be sure the flap would not be too small.

The probe of the doppler ultrasound was passed gently across the skin of Chance's thigh. "Whoosh, whoosh, whoosh" indicated the pulse and the position of two skin perforators. Their positions were marked on the skin, and the template was then positioned with one perforator centered on the skin paddle for the mouth, and another perforator centered on the skin paddle for the cheek.

At 7:50 a.m., along with Andrew P., the plastic surgery resident, I began to simultaneously harvest the ALT free flap and a latissimus free flap. The latissimus flap would be used to replace the tissue missing behind and above the left ear. The left neck was unbruised without bite wounds. Our scalpel made a gently curving incision through the neck separating the muscles, nerves, and lymph nodes surrounding the vessels. The multiple arterial branches of the external carotid artery and the small veins draining back into the internal jugular vein were dissected completely free from the surrounding tissue. Compared to adults, the external carotid artery in children often is positioned higher in the neck, more underneath the mandible. Vascular loops, small silicone strings, were passed around the external carotid artery. With these in place, the carotid was retracted out of the depths of the neck from underneath the mandible, allowing greater visualization of the vessels, making the microsurgical anastomoses technically easier. Four microvascular anastomoses were done: one artery and one vein for each flap. The vessel loops were released. Both flaps instantaneously began to bleed with normal blood flow. Skin grafts were then harvested from the posterior thigh to cover the exposed latissimus muscle and to replace the skin ripped off the eyelids. At 3:13 a.m. the following day, 19 hours and 23 minutes later, after three nursing and anesthesiology shifts, the operation was concluded. The resident and I went to the call room to catch a few hours of sleep.

Chance was taken back to the ICU. Balloons and "Happy Birthday" signs greeted Chance as he returned to the ICU. It was his 10th birthday.

The near entire skull and forehead still needed reconstruction. To protect the bone from drying out, we covered the skull with wet, sterile gauze, and we began to plan the next operation. Bone denuded of any tissue, such as all layers of the scalp, will not accept a skin graft unless the bone is first covered with vascularized tissue. A skin graft does not have its own blood supply; thus, it must be placed on top of tissue that is well perfused. Blood vessels from this tissue then grow into the skin graft to allow it to heal.

Prior to free tissue transfer, a common method to allow bone to accept a skin graft was to drill the outer layer of the bone off until the bone began to bleed. Then with time, this bleeding bone will develop new tissue, called granulation tissue. Granulation tissue is new connective tissue that appears as red, bumpy tissue. It is highly vascular. For large wounds it can take weeks to months for enough granulation tissue to develop to cover a wound. Infection, lack of moisture, minor trauma such as bumping the area, and poor wound care can prevent granulation tissue from becoming robust or confluent enough to accept a skin graft. Importantly, drilling off the outer table of the skull can also put the bone at risk for osteomyelitis and lead to intracranial infections, brain infections, which can be life-threatening.

The transfer of a free flap to the skull decreases these risks and allows the quickest, most reliable method for healing. However, putting a free flap on top of the head is not easy. The first challenge is determining what blood supply can be used to reestablish blood supply to the flap. The vessels in front of the ear, the superficial temporal artery and vein, are the nearest. Without these vessels, one has to go to the neck and to other branches from the carotid artery, internal jugular vein, and/or the external jugular vein. To reach the neck, the flap must have a pedicle that is long enough to extend from the skull to the neck, or vein grafts must first be attached to the vessels in the neck and then tunneled to the head, to the site of the reconstruction.

The second challenge is to determine which flap has the surface area large enough to reconstruct the defect. The largest muscle flap and the largest skin flap in the body are respectively a latissimus and an ALT free flap. The omentum is a large apron-like fold of tissue, mainly fatty tissue (i.e., visceral peritoneum), that hangs down from the stomach. It can be harvested as a free flap by dissecting its blood supply, the gastro-epiploic vessels off the stomach. In addition to its potential immense surface area (with a range varying greatly from approximately 300 cm^2 to 1,500 cm^2 in adults), it has a long vascular pedicle. The principal limitation of the use of an omental free flap is the need for laporatomy, which can uncommonly lead to complications, such as abdominal hernia or injury to the intra-abdominal organs.

Three days after the first major reconstruction, Chance was brought back to the operating room. Chance's bare skull stared at us; it served as a reminder of mortality. One simply cannot live with the top of their head skinned. Measuring began again. The anticipated dimensions of the remaining lattisimus muscle on the left were drawn on a towel. It covered maybe half of the skull and missing forehead. A second ALT free flap from the other leg would also be too small. What about dissecting deeper into the armpit to obtain other muscles of the chest wall and skin of the back? The blood supply of some of this combined tissue had a common source, named the sub-scapular artery and vein. A mega-flap containing the lattisimus muscle, serratus muscle, and skin overlying the scapula could be harvested. Another template was drawn, but this did not quite fit. Where Chance needed tissue, the various components of this mega-flap did not reach. Moreover, no vessels remained on the left side of the face and neck which could provide a blood supply to a new flap. Any additional anastomoses would have to go to the right. Vein grafts would be needed to extend the blood supply from the right neck to the top of the head. This left only the omental free flap as a possible single option that could cover the massive defect.

A laparotomy was done. We reached into the belly and gently eviscerated the omentum and the stomach until they laid on top of the abdominal wall spread out like a peacock's feathers. The omentum was broad but thin, with little fat. You could see through it like a transparent curtain. This was not going to work, to be able to completely cover the skull, to be thick enough to accept a skin graft, but we had already made the laparotomy and entered the abdomen. We had just harmed, possibly with no benefit. An awful feeling filled my gut. At this point you have to clear your mind, step back, and reformulate a new plan. We put the omentum and stomach back into the abdomen and covered the opening with a warm, moist towel.

There is a rough correlation between the size of the omentum and a patient's height and weight. However, in any individual it is still hard to predict. Chance's omentum could cover some of the skull and be thick enough if folded on itself. Thus, perhaps, it could still be used to some advantage. A second flap would be needed, but that meant additional micro-vascular anastomoses. At least one more artery and vein would need to be connected, and there was not a blood supply without vein grafts. Vein grafts introduce an extra element of risk. They are dissected out of the body, usually from the lower leg beginning on the foot or around the ankle. The dissection stops when you have obtained enough length to reach, to bridge the divide between the chosen vessel in the neck and the site where the pedicle of the flap rests on top of the head. How it is handled as you dissect, how the diameter of the graft compares to the diameter of the vessel in the pedicle, and how they are positioned when transferred, hopefully without a twist or kink, can predispose them to form a blood clot. There is no blood flow to the flap with a clot; there is only a dead flap.

Microsurgical expertise is all about knowing how to preserve and create blood supply. Importantly, I had also been trained first as an otolaryngologist – head and neck surgeon and then completed an additional fellowship in head and neck oncology, before I began my plastic surgery residency. Radiation therapy is a standard treatment for many patients with head and neck cancer. With a recurrence after radiation therapy, a patient will often need an extensive resection of the involved tissue, often of the mandible, tongue, and/or facial skin. These patients likely have had a previous neck dissection to remove the lymph nodes to which the cancer may have metastasized. The surgeon may have few vessels in the neck to which he can sew his flap. These vessels are typically tied off during the neck dissection and/or may be encased in scar from the previous radiation therapy. In other words, the neck has been "vessel depleted". Finding one artery and one vein in a neck that is relatively depleted is still usually possible. However, for massive defects where two free flaps are needed, this can be insurmountable.

Older techniques, reminiscent of Gillies's "Tubed Pedicle" flaps, can be used to rotate flaps from the chest or the back into the mouth, face, or neck without the need for microsurgery. However, more elegant solutions can also be devised. One technique that is occasionally used, particularly in the "vessel depleted neck", is called a "flow-through flap".[3–5] With this technique, the pedicles of two separate free flaps are sewn together; the distal end of the pedicle for the first free flap serves as the blood supply to a second free flap. Blood flows from the recipient vessels, usually branches of the external carotid artery and internal jugular vein, through the pedicle of the first free flap and into the pedicle of the second free flap. In general, there are three free flaps in the human body which can be designed as flow-through flaps. These are a fibular free flap, a RFFF, and an ALT. Maybe we could salvage Chance's omental flap using the "flow-through" technique?

In complex reconstruction, you often do not know whether a course of action is going to be successful until you have tried. Previous experience and confidence in yourself, perhaps misguided, will bias your estimate of the probability of success and how you describe a procedure to a patient. For the patient, a surgical consent for a complex reconstruction is never 100% informed. The surgeon does his best to explain all of the risks, options, and benefits so that the patient can decide accordingly with the surgeon. However, every step in microsurgery depends on the previous step, and the outcome of each step leads to a different option. The blood supply to the flap that is revealed intra-operatively, the diameter of the blood vessels, and multiple other anatomic considerations will determine how you proceed. Patient characteristics, such as weight, age, previous scars, and activity level, affect how you choose and design a flap.

Chance is an active young boy who likes to play soccer. Should I avoid taking any flap from his legs? For this particular patient, is there a better flap? How do you define "better"? The potential plan becomes a massive decision tree with probabilities and different outcomes. You, as the treating surgeon, outline this thought process to the patient and the family. Ultimately, the informed consent relies on trust. They trust that you have thoroughly considered every outcome, including the harm/morbidity that your reconstruction will introduce. They trust that you can deliver what you envision, but the crystal ball is always cloudy.

With the omentum waiting in the abdomen, it was decided to harvest a right ALT free flap and to try to use the "flow-through" technique to perfuse the omentum as a second free flap. The omentum was delivered back onto the abdomen wall. The short gastric vessels connecting the omentum to the greater curvature of the stomach were taken down. The flap was left pedicled on the right gastroepiploic artery and vein, bunched together to provide greater thickness, and then measured. With a bunched surface area now only 15 cm x 10 cm, it could cover only, maybe, one-third of the skull. The anticipated remaining defect on the skull was measured. These measurements were then transferred to the right leg, and a massive ALT flap (26 cm x 11 cm) was designed.

For the harvest, the medial skin incision on the thigh was first made. The fascia deep to the skin on top of the quadricep muscles was lifted to confirm the position and presence of the perforators that had been heard with a Doppler probe through the skin. Though two had been heard, only one perforator was found perfusing the skin. This could be a problem; without multiple perforators perfusing such a large piece of tissue, the tissue could die, becoming necrotic farther away from the perforator. However, the skin edges on the very end of the flap, farthest away from the perforator, bled bright red when rubbed. We decided to proceed, basing the entire flap on the one perforator. At least for now, perfusion seemed adequate. There was no other option.

Once tissue is taken out of the body, with its blood supply divided, it immediately begins to slowly die. It is acutely ischemic; damage begins to occur to the microcirculation and cells within the flap. Tissue can tolerate acute ischemia for a certain period of time. This is why placing a tourniquet or inflating a blood pressure cuff for a few minutes to momentarily stop blood flow to an extremity causes no harm. If a blood vessel is intentionally divided, as is done during the transfer of a free flap, or is obstructed by a clot, revascularization and restoration of blood supply must be achieved as soon as possible to prevent irreversible damage. However, not all tissue demonstrates equal susceptibility to ischemia. For free tissue transfer, the omentum and jejunum have the shortest ischemia times, referenced in textbooks to be between 2 and 4 hours. After this critical threshold, even if the artery and vein have been reconnected, the cellular damage that has occurred in the tissue of the flap is so extensive that the tissue of the flap dies. Muscle (i.e., such as of the latissimus and gracilis muscles) has the next shortest ischemia of between 4 and 6 hours, followed by skin and bone.

With both the omentum and the ALT flap still attached to their blood supply, respectively in the abdomen and the leg, anticipating ischemia time now became critical. It must be minimized. The recipient vessels must be prepared so that when the flap is brought to the site needing reconstruction, there is little left to do except to sew the vessels together under the microscope. If set up properly, the anastomoses should take about 30–40 minutes for both the artery and vein. For Chance, the nearest remaining blood vessels were the right superficial temporal artery and vein in front of the ear, but these were still 8 centimeters away from where the pedicle of the ALT flap would lie once the flap had been set into the scalp defect.

The legs were examined for vein grafts. To save Chance's life, the right greater saphenous vein, just above the ankle, had been used for multiple intravenous infusions of fluid and blood when he arrived in the emergency room. Multiple needle sticks had made this vein unusable. Therefore, with an incision going from the ankle into the midcalf, the left greater saphenous vein was harvested. The vein graft was then divided into two pieces, sewn to the STA and STV, and placed at the top of the head next to where the ALT flap was to be inset (Figure 2.4). Now we were ready to divide the blood supply, the pedicle of the ALT free flap.

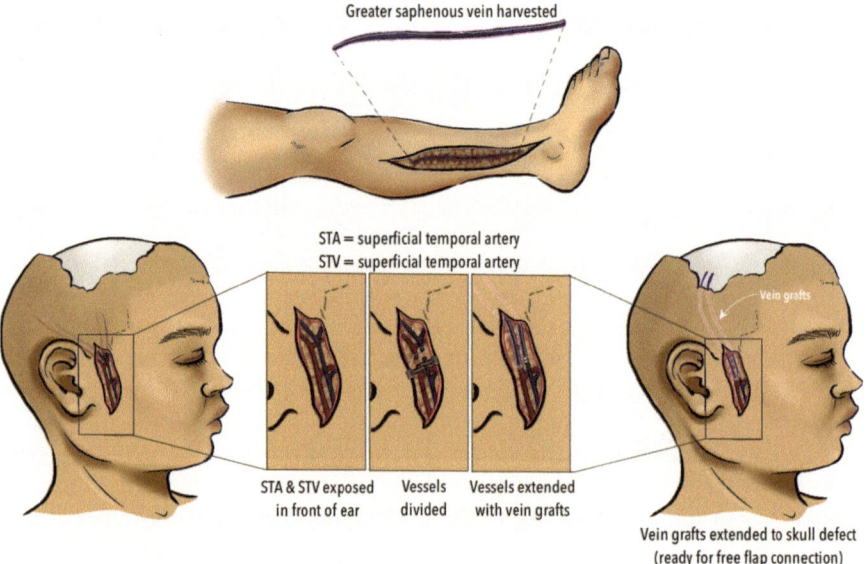

Greater saphenous vein harvested

STA = superficial temporal artery
STV = superficial temporal artery

Vein grafts

STA & STV exposed   Vessels   Vessels extended
in front of ear   divided   with vein grafts

Vein grafts extended to skull defect
(ready for free flap connection)

Figure 2.4 Scalp defect with vessel selection and vein grafts for placing a blood supply on top of the head – defect from lateral view.

The greater saphenous vein from the left leg was harvested as a vein graft (Upper Panel). It was divided into 2 segments and then sewn into the 2 normal vessels in front of the ear (i.e., the Superficial Temporal Artery and Vein [STA and STV]). The connected vein grafts were then tunneled underneath the scalp to reach the top of the head where the scalp was missing (Lower Panel). The ALT free flap would then be connected to these grafts.

Thirty-five minutes later, the ALT was successfully anastomosed to the two vein grafts leading back to the STA and STV. The lateral descending circumflex artery (LDCA) and vein (LDCV), the axial blood supply which sends the perforators to the skin paddle of the ALT, were examined. There was a robust pulse within the flap, and all of the skin edges were now bleeding with bright red blood. The small vascular clamps on the distal ends of the LDCA and LDCV, past the proximal anastomoses to the vein grafts, were released, and blood shot across the skull.

The distal end of the ALT's pedicle was ready for the second free flap. The microscope was repositioned. The omentum was divided from the stomach. Thirty minutes later, the omentum was pink and bleeding on top of the skull (Figure 2.5). At 2:30 a.m., after being in the operating room for 19 hours, Chance rejoined his parents in the ICU with his skull now completely covered with well-perfused tissue (Figure 2.6).

A pediatric ICU transforms itself during Christmas week. It becomes a place of joy with glowing Christmas trees, visits from Santa, and nurses dressed as elves. Sedation and the intrusion of the ventilator clouded any hope that Chance would participate in any meaningful way in this celebration. Chance was now also 6 days from his last surgery, a time when I knew that we would see just how good the perfusion was going to be on the edges of the ALT flap. Circumferentially around the edges of the flap, farthest away from the single perforator, the skin was no longer pink but gray. These areas did not

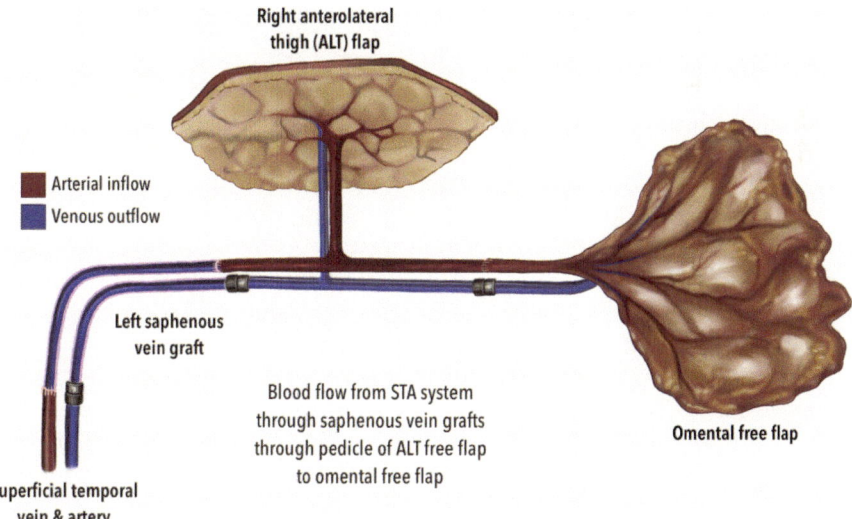

Figure 2.5 "Flow-through" technique for perfusing two free flaps in series.

The omental free flap was perfused by a "flow-through" technique connecting the pedicle of the ALT free flap to the pedicle of the omental free flap. Blood flows through the first free flap into a second free flap.

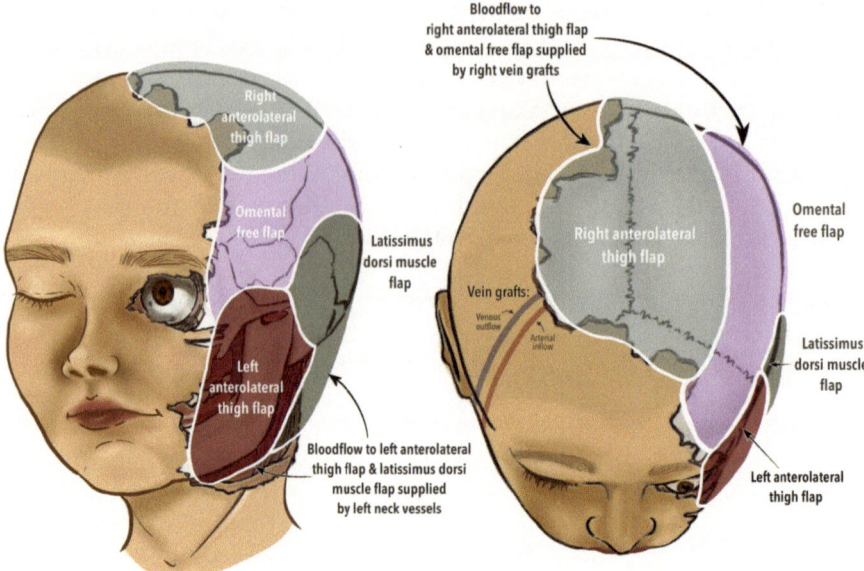

Figure 2.6 Chance's reconstruction with four free flaps.

Using multiple vein grafts and the "flow-through" technique, two ante-rolateral thigh free flaps, an omental free flap, and a latissimus free flap were used to replace the missing tissue of the face and scalp.

bleed when pricked with a small needle. This tissue was dead and needed to be removed, and this needed to be done soon. The pedicle of the reattached omental free flap was under this dead tissue, and this would eventually lead to infection, clotting, and blood flow obstruction to this flap.

Urgently, Chance was taken back to the operating room. With a knife and scissors, the dead edges of the ALT free flap were cut away. The remaining half of the original ALT flap was picked up and moved over to cover the pedicle of the omental free flap. Could this be called a success? The flaps were still alive; 75% of the original skull defect was now covered with vas-cularized tissue. However, with the debridement and the repositioning, the bone of the left skull was now again fully exposed.

Sleep fragmented by worries about your patients is inevitable if you are doing complex operations with risk. In your dreams, you watch your hands move, tie knots, and reposition the microscope. Elaborate decision trees devised to solve a problem crowd out any other thoughts. You might try to pull yourself out of sleep, to wake yourself, to write down an idea before it disappears into a forgotten dream.

Eight hours later, I received an emergent page from the ICU that knocked me out of sleep back into the present. Chance now had a "blown right pupil" and was not moving the left side of his body. Nothing that I had done or had anticipated should have put Chance's brain at risk for a stroke. He was emergently whisked down to the radiology department to obtain a CT and MRI scan to check on perfusion to his brain.

Outside the scanner, I did one last check on the flaps. With a doppler over the pedicles, there was no sound, no pulse. For some reason, the flaps now had no perfusion. They were both now ischemic with imminent death, and we could do nothing until we understood if the brain was being perfused and needed treatment. One hour later, the scans revealed normal perfusion to the brain. Chance was beginning to move his left leg. Perhaps, a cerebral vessel had gone into spasm and was now relaxed, allowing normal blood flow. The neurosurgical team agreed that it was safe to take Chance back to the operating room. Irreversible tissue death, caused by a prolonged ischemia time, was now a real possibility.

The skin sutures overlying the site of the vein grafts were removed. The vein graft going from the STA into the LDCA was completely clotted. With scissors I cut the anastomosis in half, and blood immediately shot out of the STA. Compression from turning the head, maybe a mismatch in vessel size between the vein graft and the other vessels, had caused the clot. Quickly, Chance's right leg was prepped with Betadine to harvest another vein graft. My own movements seemed to be slowed by my frequent glances at the clock to calculate the ever-increasing ischemia time. The resident picked up the leg and held it laterally rotated so we could quickly harvest the lesser saphenous vein located on the posterior aspect of the calf.

Forty-five minutes later, the new vein graft was completely connected. Flow from the superficial temporal artery now proceeded through the lesser saphenous vein graft, through the lateral descending circumflex artery, and though the right gastro-epiploic artery. The skin of the ALT flap and the mucosa and fat of the omental flap were pink. Total estimated Ischemia time: 5 hours, 17 minutes. Contrary to the textbook teaching about ischemia, both flaps were alive and well.

For the remaining hospitalization, Chance's free flaps remained well perfused. The bone that was exposed on the left skull was drilled down and cared for with dressing changes in the operating room every 4–5 days for the next 3 months, a total of 15 additional operations, until they were ready to accept skin grafts. On the 90th day after the dog attack, Chance, dressed as a superhero (Figure 2.7), left the hospital.

Since his return to his hometown, Chance has thrived with the assistance of his parents and an abundance of goodwill from his community. After his return home, Chance's elementary school and Budget Way, a used car dealership in his town, held fundraisers for Chance and raised a total of about $3,600. The local high school at the behest of Chance's older brother, a freshman, held another fundraiser. The high school play production of *Cinderella* raised about $1,500 for Chance, who attended three of the four shows and appeared onstage with the actors and crew members to give a

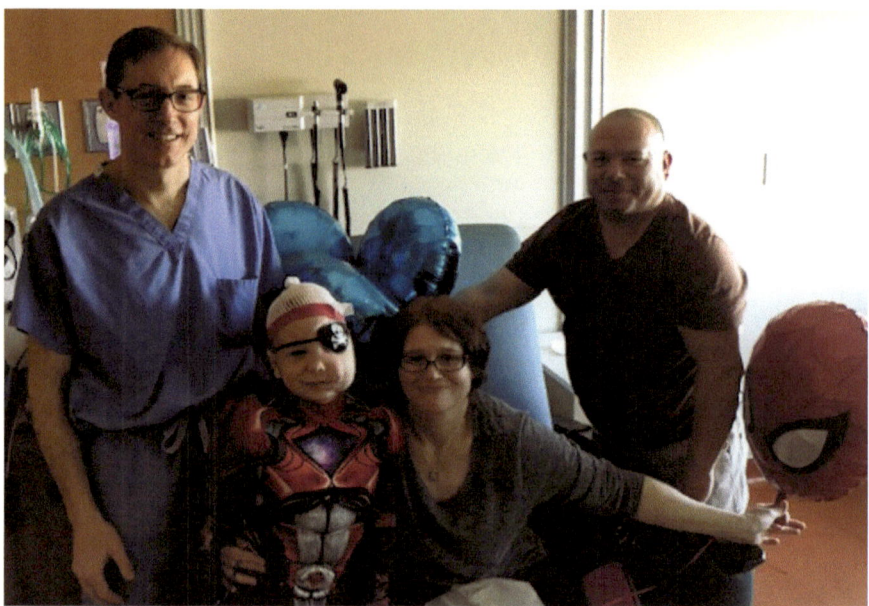

Figure 2.7 Chance and his family on the day of discharge.

Dressed as superhero, Chance left the hospital 3 months after his trauma. As a high school student he is an Honor Student and State Champion in bowling.

bow to the audience at the end. Chance's GoFundMe account generated $7,112 from 123 donations.

In the immediate months and years after completion of his surgeries, Chance maintained a youthful exuberance. In middle school he became an honors student and, in his mother's words, "quite a charmer", with a close group of friends. His brother commented that "every once in a while he gets pretty down when we're alone, thinking, 'Oh, no one's going to like me because of how I look'". However, Chance's family reassures him that people will always love him for who he is, regardless of anything else.

As a junior in high school as of this writing, Chance has continued to excel academically and socially. He has earned the distinction of an "A Honor Roll Student" for multiple, consecutive years and helped lead his high school bowling team to a state bowling championship in 2023.[6] I asked his mom, now more than 6 years after the injury, "Why do you think Chance has had such strength and success after his accident?" Her response: "When people ask what happened here? Chance simply states, it happened; deal with it. He is doing great because he has moved past his injury".

The psychological and body image effects of facial trauma on quality of life have been extensively studied. Even with minor trauma, such as an isolated facial laceration or facial fracture, when compared with a control population, a group of individuals who have suffered facial trauma often have a statistically significant lower satisfaction with life, increase in depression, more negative perception of body image, and a higher incidence of post-traumatic stress disorder, unemployment, alcoholism, and marital problems.

Support and encouragement from family and community undoubtedly aid in recovery. But can this recovery ever be psychologically complete, especially in a devasting injury such as Chance's? The public will always be able to see, and will react, to the scars of his trauma and reconstruction. How will Chance interpret and internalize these reactions? For any given patient, this is impossible to predict. I have seen patients, my own patients, who have suffered gunshot wounds, some of them self-inflected, with reconstructed faces who present years after the injury for follow-up. They are dressed in their work clothes and often accompanied by their significant other. They chat about their children and how they look forward to their upcoming ski season or school year. However, others simply disappear after they are released from the hospital. They are unable to be reached by phone.

Gillies recognized how severe disfigurement can handicap a person for life. Some of his patients never left the Queen's Hospital, unwilling to re-enter a possible hostile world. In the 1950s, one of the nurses at Queen Mary's Hospital Sidcup lamented:

> We had two night watchmen, both wounded very badly in WWI. They had gone through facial reconstructive procedures after the War, but the price they paid for their Country was unbelievable. They were so disfigured, only night work was possible; they never looked us in the face, but we (the nurses) began to feel comfortable with them, feed them a sandwich and a cup of tea on a cold night ... Stan the one I knew the best told me he had never had a family, never been to a dance, never enjoyed a girlfriend even before the war.[7]

Years ago, I spent the majority of my academic research time studying the quality of life (QOL) of patients with head and neck cancer.[7–12] At the University of Washington (UW), under the guidance of Ernest Weymuller, MD, Chair of the Department of Otolaryngology, we studied how patients were affected psychologically and functionally by their treatment, including by their reconstruction with free flaps. We wrote and validated one of the standard QOL indexes, the UW QOL measure, that is still widely used to evaluate QOL. The original UW QOL index was a disease-specific questionnaire that focuses on measuring function in 12 domains: pain, appearance, activity, recreation, swallowing, chewing, speech, shoulder, taste, saliva, mood, and anxiety. Each domain was also given a score which scaled its relative importance in relation to the other domains. For example, for a particular patient, the absence or control of pain may be more important than the ability to speak well or return to a normal diet.

With multiple publications and through interviews with hundreds of patients, we revealed some important truths. First, over time, often as a consequence of treatment, patients often change the priorities of what is important in their lives. For example, speech and swallowing after treatment could become more important than appearance compared to before treatment. Second, even though a treatment can be disfiguring, patients often did not report this as important. The surgeon may place greater importance on appearance than the patient. This became clear when we followed 10 patients who underwent a laryngectomy (i.e., removal of the voice box) for cancer of the larynx.[9] Two years post-surgery and without evidence of recurrent cancer, we found that post-laryngectomy total QOL was not significantly different from the pre-larygnectomy scores. In all QOL domains, including speech and appearance, 50% or more of the patients reported having the same or better function at 2 years post-treatment. We also found that although loss of speech was disabling and a laryngectomy was disfiguring, only a minority of patients reported speech or appearance as being more than "somewhat important". They indicated that "activity" (i.e., socialization) was the most important issue. Being alive and with family was of extreme importance.

The supplemental comments of patients confirmed that the majority had maintained a good to excellent overall QOL even after disfiguring surgery. One patient's quote summarized this sentiment:

> I enjoy getting up in the morning, still going to work and getting out for an occasional round of golf with my sons and grandson. Also, my sex life has recently taken a turn for the better.[9]

What matters most is hope. If a patient feels that he has lost his future, a future of developing relationships, of being part of a community, then intense sorrow will be the only outcome that is real. Surgeons can marshal the most cutting-edge medicine to heal a patient's wound, but they play such a small role in this final long-term outcome. Hope is preserved and enhanced by those who love the patient. We can only hope that all of our patients return to a loving environment where they are protected and valued.

The patient who does the best after reconstruction is the one who does not lose who he is (i.e., his sense of identity), the one who finds or creates a bigger purpose than himself. Nic Patrick is such a patient.

On June 20, 2013, on a bright summer morning, Nic Patrick was walking along his hay fields to irrigate his fields in South Fork Valley, 22 miles west of Cody, Wyoming.[13] All of a sudden, he heard his dog screaming in pain. As he rushed around the corner of the hill, he came face to face with a female grizzly bear and her two cubs. "She looked at me about 25 yards away and basically said you're next," recalled Nic. "And she was on me in two and half seconds. She came in and swung, and I hit her on the side of the head with my shovel, and it just made her madder probably. Bit me full in the face". The bear backed off. Nic grabbed his cell phone to call for help. No service. The grizzly was not done. "I could hear her coming back huffing and puffing". She then dragged him for 20 yards by the knee. Twenty seconds later, she left, Nic said.

With his upper lip dangling and the side of this face and nose ravaged, Nic walked the quarter mile back to his ranch. His wife, Joyce, daughter, son-in-law, and four grandchildren were in the house. He stopped in the shed before entering the house to cover his face with a rag. "So I wouldn't scare the hell out of them," Nic said. A few miles outside Cody, an ambulance greeted Nic and his family. The next thing that he remembers was awaking in Denver in the ICU.

The bear had bit off a large portion of the right cheek and entire nose (Figure 2.8). At the first operation, we debrided the unhealthy tissue and fixed the facial fractures by putting the bones back in their proper places with titanium screws and plates. A week after the first surgery, we

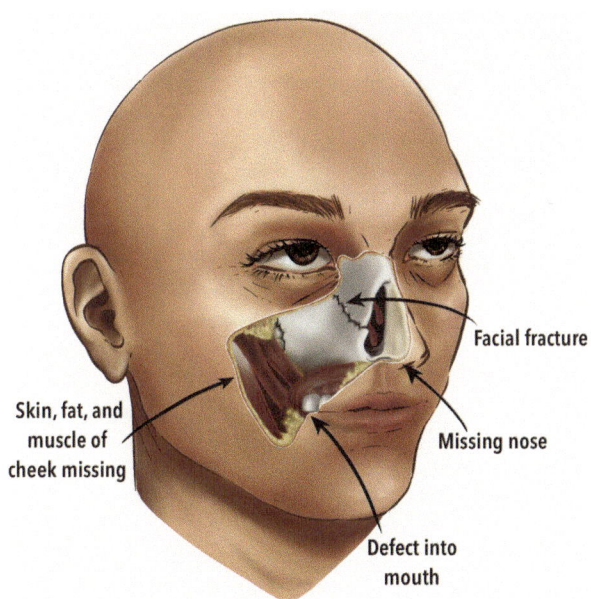

Figure 2.8 Defect created by bear attack.

A grizzly bear removed the right cheek and nose of Nic Patrick and fractured the underlying bones.

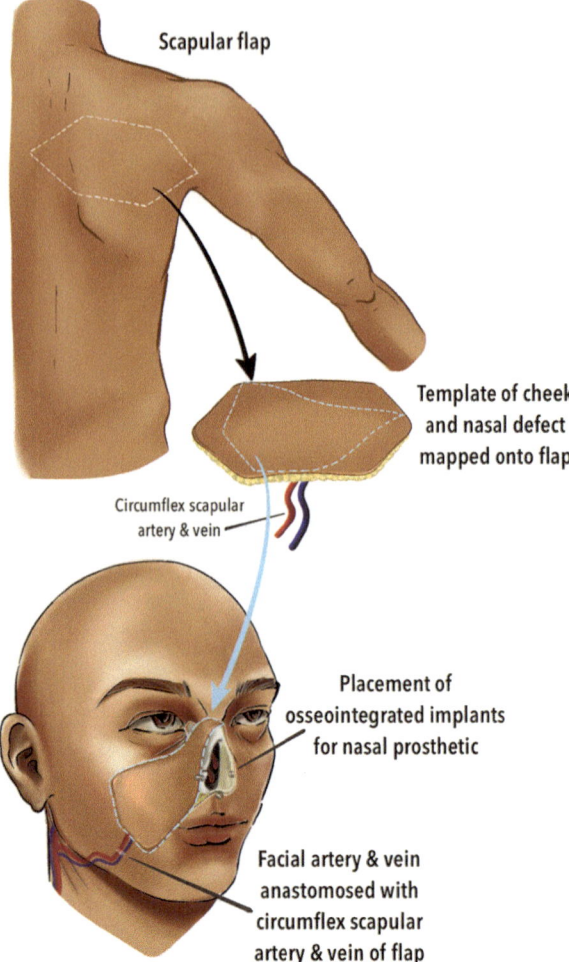

Scapular flap

Template of cheek
and nasal defect
mapped onto flap

Circumflex scapular
artery & vein

Placement of
osseointegrated implants
for nasal prosthetic

Facial artery & vein
anastomosed with
circumflex scapular
artery & vein of flap

Figure 2.9 Scapular flap used for cheek reconstruction.

A scapular flap harvested from the back was used to reconstruct the right cheek. Screws with a post (i.e., osteo-integrated implants, similar to what is used for dental implants) were placed into the bones around the nose so that a nasal prosthetic could be worn.

undertook the second. A template of the missing cheek was outlined. Nic was then rolled onto his side. The template was transferred to Nic's back in order to harvest a scapular free flap, containing the skin, fat, and fascia around Nic's shoulder blade (Figure 2.9). With the flap harvested, Nic was placed back into a supine (lying flat) position, and the scapular free flap was sewn into vessels of the face. The scapular free tissue transfer laid the groundwork for the subsequent three 1- to-2-hour, outpatient operations that were done to thin and contour the flap tissue to restore Nic's natural appearance to the greatest extent possible. As Nic told me, "Dr. D., we have spent a lot of quality time together."[14]

Nic was still missing his entire nose. A total nasal reconstruction can be done with a combination of a free flap, rib grafts, and a pedicled forehead flap, but the reconstruction requires multiple stages and months of surgery. Nic opted for a nasal prosthetic. Therefore, in 2015 we placed osteo-integrated implants, similar to what is placed for dental implants, within the reconstructed bone of the midface. With magnets, the nasal prosthetic now attaches to these implants. As Nic says, "unless someone looks really close, they do not know my nose is missing." Kudos to Barbara Spohn-Lillo, board-certified clinical anaplastologist, who made Nic's nasal prosthesis with precise detail to match his skin tone, blend with his scars, and replicate his natural nose from pre-trauma photographs.

Initially, Nic blamed himself for not being careful enough. He had seen grizzlies in the area the day before the attack. Later, he realized that he was "damned lucky to be alive". Nic even laments that the grizzlies will be blamed for the attack. He was in their habitat. The sow was just protecting her cubs.

For 40 years, Nic, a Greater Yellowstone Coalition member, had advocated protecting the grizzlies and the ecosystem. His near brush has not changed his stance for the grizzlies and protecting other wildlife in Yellowstone. He states that "what is key is protecting the wild places animals inhabit from development for future generations of humans to treasure".

Patrick commends the medical staff for his care, his children for running the business while he was in the hospital, and his neighbors for taking care of the hay in his absence. His wife, Joyce, deserves the most credit. "She basically saved my life. I couldn't have made this recovery without her support and encouragement", he said. "I went through the stages that happen when you lose someone," Nic said. "I went through a couple of hours of 'Why me?'" He continues to live his life with his loving family, promoting the causes in which he believes. "I didn't lose anything that I couldn't live without", such as family members or his life. "It's just surface damage", he said. "I want somebody to learn something from it".

Indeed, thousands have read and heard Nic's story. In May 2016, *National Geographic* published a special issue highlighting the battle between wildlife and humans in Yellowstone National Park.[15] Nic was featured in a 2-page, center photograph- his reconstructed face fully visible, casting no blame or regret (Figure 2.10). A 4-minute video telling his story was posted on the *National Geographic* website. As Nic says, "Life isn't about what you get, but what you make of it".

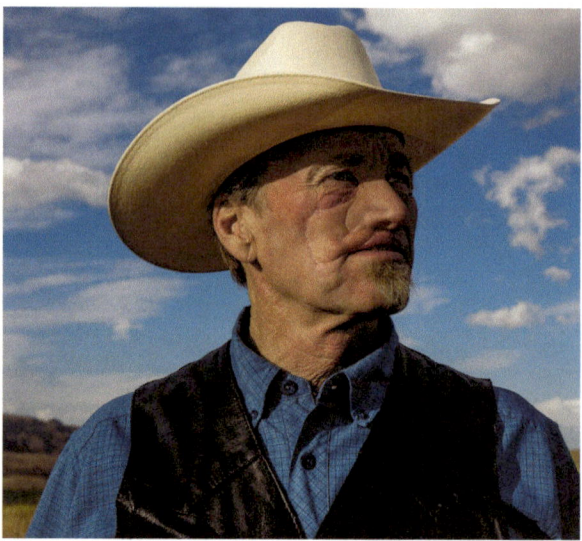

Figure 2.10 Final reconstruction of Nic Patrick.

Image published in *National Geographic Magazine*, 2016.

REFERENCES

1. Gillies HD, Millard DR. *The Principles and Art of Plastic Surgery*. Little, Brown and Company, 1957, pp. 45–46.
2. Londberg M. Kansas boy survives a gruesome attack by his neighbor's dog but faces a long recovery. *The Kansas City Star*, January 4, 2018 (https://www.kansascity.com>local>article192954844).
3. Rodriguez IE, Trinh BB, Deleyiannis FW. Utility of an anterior tibial perforator for skin paddle viability in through-and-through defects of the Mandible. *Eplasty*. 2018 Sep 20;18:e24.
4. Sokoya M, Deleyiannis FW. A triple pedicle, near-total thigh flap supercharged with the Flow-through technique. *Eplasty*. 2016 Jan 13;16:e4.
5. Trinh BB, French B, Khechoyan DY, Deleyiannis FW. Designing a fibular flow-through flap with a proximal peroneal perforator-free flap for maxillary reconstruction. *Plast Reconstr Surg Glob Open*. 2017 Nov 7;5(11):e1543.
6. Maycock B. Happy place yields state championship as Garden State shocks coach with Unified Bowling title. *KSHSAA Covered*, November 14, 2023 (https://kshsaacovered.com/news/2023/11/14/boys-bowling-happy-place-yields-state-championship-as-garden-city-shocks-coach-with-unified-bowling-title.aspx).
7. https://www.nam.ac.uk/the-birth-of-plastic-surgery.
8. Weymuller EA Jr, Yueh B, Deleyiannis FW, Kuntz AL, Alsarraf R, Coltrera MD. Quality of life in head and neck cancer. *Laryngoscope*. 2000 Mar;110(3 Pt 3):4–7.

9. Deleyiannis FW, Weymuller EA Jr, Coltrera MD, Futran N. Quality of life after laryngectomy: are functional disabilities important? *Head Neck*. 1999 Jul;21(4):319–324.

10. Deleyiannis FW, Weymuller EA Jr, Coltrera MD. Quality of life of disease-free survivors of advanced (stage III or IV) oropharyngeal cancer. *Head Neck*. 1997 Sep;19(6):466–473.

11. Weymuller EA Jr, Alsarraf R, Yueh B, Deleyiannis FW, Coltrera MD. Analysis of the performance characteristics of the University of Washington Quality of Life instrument and its modification (UW-QOL-R). *Arch Otolaryngol Head Neck Surg*. 2001 May;127(5):489–493.

12. Weymuller EA, Yueh B, Deleyiannis FW, Kuntz AL, Alsarraf R, Coltrera MD. Quality of life in patients with head and neck cancer: lessons learned from 549 prospectively evaluated patients. *Arch Otolaryngol Head Neck Surg*. 2000 Mar;126(3):329–335; discussion 335–336.

13. Mathers G. South Fork man gravely injured by grizzly. *Powell Tribune*, June 25, 2013 (https://powelltribune.com/stories/south-fork-man-gravely-injured-by-grizzly,5577).

14. Smith T. Wyoming man's face rebuilt at University of Colorado after grizzly attack. *CU Anschutz Newsroom*, April 9, 2015 (https://news.cuanschutz.edu/news-stories/Wyoming-man's-face-rebuilt-at-University-of-Colorado-after-grizzly-attack).

15. America's Wild West idea Yellowstone. *National Geographic* (Yellowstone: The Battle for the American West). 2016 May;229(5):48–49.

Chapter 3

Limb salvage

Is all this worthwhile?

> Your state of your life is nothing more than a reflection of the state of your mind.
>
> – Wayne W. Dyer, 1940–2015
> *American self-help author and motivational speaker*

An amputation is a radical and irreversible intervention. In the United States, vascular insufficiency to the lower limbs from peripheral vascular disease (PVD) and/or from diabetes mellitus-related vasculopathy is the leading indication for an amputation. The reason for an amputation varies from country to country and from regions within the same country. Smoking, obesity, and hypertension increase the risk of PVD. Post-traumatic gangrene, chronic osteomyelitis (i.e., infection of the underlying bone), and malignancy can be an indication for an amputation.

Severe trauma can also be an indication. With extremity trauma, the severity of the injury is based on evaluating four functional components: bones and joints, soft tissues, vessels, and nerves. Limbs are considered "mangled "with injury to three of these four elements. Presently, from all causes in the United States, about 30,000 to 40,000 amputations are done annually. The vast majority are from the lower extremity.

Historically, war trauma was the main indication for an amputation. Of the approximate 60,000 operations done during the American Civil War (1861–1865), it has been estimated that three-quarters of these were amputations, done mainly to prevent complications, in particular life-threatening infections. To assist the vast number of amputees, the federal government between 1861 and 1873 issued almost 150 patents for designs of artificial limbs. To Union veterans, $75 was allocated to buy an artificial leg and $50 for an arm.[1]

In the 1870s, Joseph Lister was instrumental in introducing the concepts of sanitation in a medical setting and the use of carbolic acid (phenol) as the first widely used antiseptic. Lister would sterilize the surgical instruments and operating room with phenol, and even soak bandages in the phenol to dress wounds. However, the incidence of amputations as a result of infections remained high, estimated to be as high as 75% of the cases in World

DOI: 10.1201/9781003538028-4

War I. In 1928 Alexander Fleming discovered the first antibiotic, but it took over a decade before penicillin was introduced as a treatment for bacterial infections.

The adoption of principles of antiseptic surgery and increasing availability of antibiotics contributed to the decreasing need for amputations during the first half of the 20th century. However, advances in the treatment of vascular injuries remained relatively dormant and continued to be a leading reason for an amputation. During World War II (1939–1945), the official policy of the Army Medical Department was that all arterial injuries should be ligated, tied off, not repaired.[2] This recommendation originated from a review of 2,471 arterial wounds, done by Colonel Michael DeBakey, Special Consultant to the Office of the Surgeon General. An amputation rate of greater than 50% was noted in those patients who underwent an attempt of arterial reconstruction with vein grafts or vitallium tubes. This rate of amputation was similar to those who simply underwent ligation of the arterial bleeders. Fine suture, delicate non-crushing clamps, and reliable (i.e., not prone to clotting) grafts had yet to be developed.

During the Korean War (1950–1953) the systematic repair of vascular injuries was introduced. This clinical experience was gained mainly in the Mobile Army Surgical Hospital (MASH) facilities, particularly after Brigadier General Holmes Ginn, Surgeon to the Eighth Army, sent an order to the MASH units that each MASH unit send two surgeons for vascular training to the 53rd Surgical Hospital (formerly 8055 MASH).[3] An additional military order instructed the collection of stray dogs so that they could be used for surgical practice. Each surgeon preformed 4–8 vascular repairs on the animals' extremities before they returned to their MASH units. Though the rates of amputation in patients with vascular injuries markedly decreased, what remained a difficult decision was whether to amputate an extremity when there was associated loss of bone, muscle, and/or nerve with a compromised circulation. The circulation could perhaps be restored with arterial reconstruction, but with an open wound, neither the fractured bone nor the vascular repair was guaranteed to heal if the overlying skin and/or muscle was injured or missing. With a nerve injury, there could also be chronic pain or an extremity that could neither feel nor move.

Until the advent of microsurgery in the 1970s, fractured limbs mangled with overlying soft tissue loss could be treated only with local pedicled skin or muscle flaps. On the most distal part of the leg, around the ankle and lower calf, there are few nearby pedicled flaps that can be rotated. Patients would often be treated with cross-leg flaps (Figure 3.1). A section of skin would be lifted from the calf of one leg and sewn to other leg to cover the wound.[4] The legs would be bound together to prevent any movement. Similar to the technique that Gilles used for pedicled flaps from the chest to the face, a cross-leg flap would be divided once its new blood supply had been established 3 or more weeks after it been inset. In 1854 Frank H Hamilton introduced the first cross-leg flap to treat a leg ulcer.

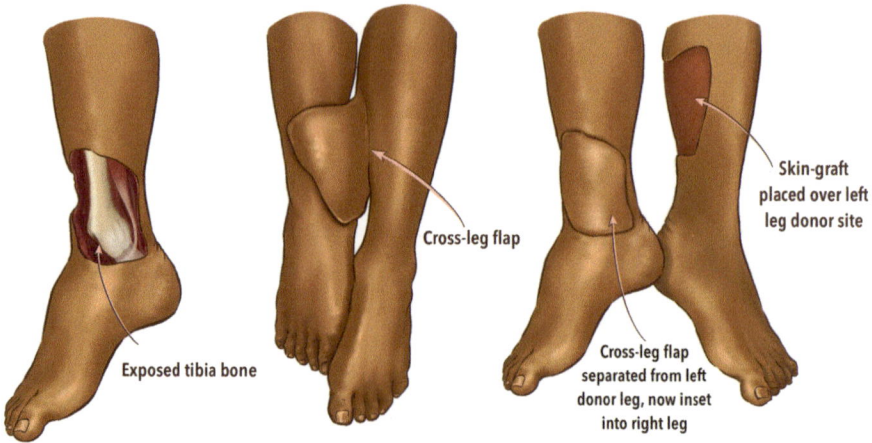

Skin-graft
placed over left
leg donor site

Cross-leg flap

Exposed tibia bone

Cross-leg flap
separated from left
donor leg, now inset
into right leg

Figure 3.1 Cross-leg flap.

Cross-leg flap used to cover exposed tibial bone. Such a flap is only done if microvascular options and/or expertise are not available.

During World War II the technique was extensively used to treat war wounds with tissue loss. The cross-leg flap is rarely used today, but it still can be a useful tool if there is no microsurgical expertise or option.

Visit a busy Level I trauma hospital today, and you will see war trauma. High-speed motor vehicle accidents, gunshot wounds, and industrial accidents crush, tear, and rip off extremities. The role of the plastic surgeon is to assist the trauma surgeon, orthopedic surgeon, and vascular surgeon in ensuring that their surgery and repairs are successful. An amputation is rarely done. If a trauma patient arrives with a completely nonviable limb attached by only a few strands of tissue, the amputation will likely be completed. In contrast, the vast majority of severely injured extremities, if we perform proper initial debridement, vascularization, and fracture stabilization, can be salvaged. Microsurgery provides the expertise to potentially treat any soft tissue loss; it has transformed the management of the mangled extremity.

On a Tuesday afternoon around 1:00 pm, Stormy, Brandon, and two of their children were traveling northbound in their black Dodge Durango on US Route 285. A Dodge Ram truck was traveling southbound. At milepost 119 at the summit of Poncha Pass, the Durango lost control on the snow-covered road and began to spin, crossing the center line into the southbound lanes. Brandon died instantaneously at the scene from the head-on collision. His two children, Konnor and Kris, were emergently transported to the Heart of Rockies Medical, the nearest medical center in Salida, Colorado. Kris, the younger brother, suffered a broken femur and lacerations to the face and scalp. Konnor was in a grave state. His right arm was shattered. Above the elbow, the humerus was in multiple bony segments; the biceps was partially missing, and no pulse was present in the forearm.[5] His blood pressure was falling, and his heart rate was racing. He was in shock.

The initial trauma evaluation, a Focused Assessment with Sonography (FAST), suggested that he was bleeding in his abdomen. He was rushed to the operating room at the Heart of Rockies. The abdomen was opened. The intestines, spleen, and liver were directly examined. No active bleeding was found. The blood loss was likely from his arm. Pins were placed into the bone above and below the fractures and connected with rods (i.e., an external fixator) to pull the arm out to its normal length, to reduce the fracture. No additional bleeding was encountered, but even with the fracture reduced, the arm was still cold and pulseless.

Extremities without a pulse are on acute ischemia time. The tissue below the arterial occlusion is not receiving any perfusion. If blood flow is not restored promptly, usually before 4–6 hours, irreversible damage will occur. Once perfusion is restored, the tissues, in particular the muscles, swell. The longer the ischemia time and the greater the crush injury, the more the muscles will swell. The muscles are divided into muscle groups by compartments of fascia, which are thick bands of connective tissue. Since these compartments are closed spaces, whenever there is any significant swelling, the muscles, vessels, and nerve are pushed against the fascia. This condition is called a compartment syndrome. The high pressure can further damage muscle and nerves and lead to further decreased blood flow. To release this pressure, one can cut the fascia (i.e., a fasciotomy) to open the closed space, to release the pressure and allow the muscles to expand. With the crush and avulsion injury that Konnor had experienced, it was just a matter of time until he developed a compartment syndrome. The surgeons in Salida performed the fasciotomies, and an emergent call went to the DocLine, a 24/7 transfer system of Memorial Hospital in Colorado Springs, the nearest Level I trauma center.

From the medical helicopter, Konner bypassed the emergency room at Memorial Hospital and went directly to the operating room. At 7:38 p.m., approximately 6 hours from the time of the injury, Dr. AK, one of the trauma surgeons, began the vascular evaluation and salvage. The right arm was prepped with Betadine, an antiseptic. The external fixator was adjusted to be sure the fracture was reduced (Figure 3.2). With the overlying biceps missing, the brachial artery, the main artery to the upper extremity, was clearly visible in the depths of the wound. Just above the site of injury, above the crushed humerus, the brachial artery could be seen beating. However, below this zone of injury where the brachial artery divides into the radial and ulnar artery, the main arterial branches to the forearm and hand, a pulse was not clearly present. Dr. AK, with a small needle, injected IV contrast into the beating brachial artery. Fluoroscopy, which provides real-time intraoperative radiographs, revealed the contrast extending through the brachial artery into the ulnar artery into the hand. There was no flow in the radial artery. The remaining muscles covering the origin of the radial and ulnar artery were retracted to the side to allow a direct visualization of the vessels.

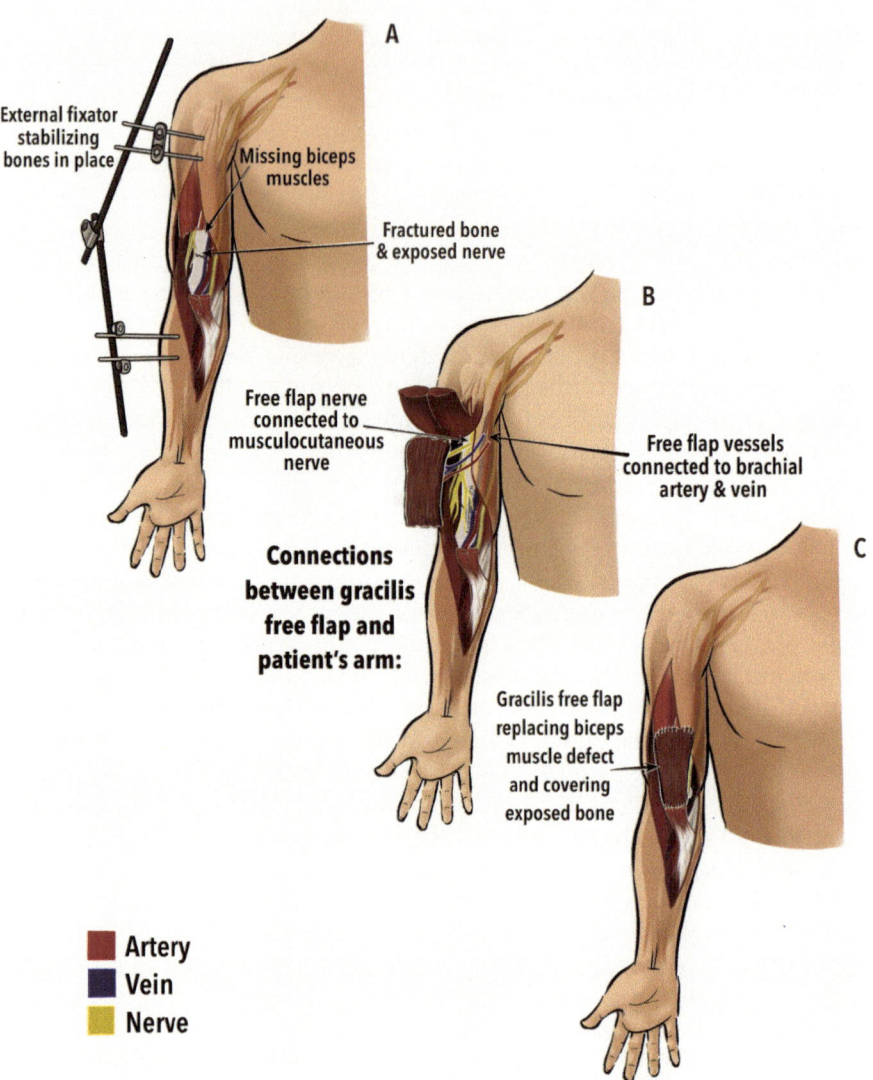

External fixator
stabilizing
bones in place

Missing biceps
muscles

Fractured bone
& exposed nerve

Free flap nerve
connected to
musculocutaneous
nerve

Free flap vessels
connected to brachial
artery & vein

**Connections
between gracilis
free flap and
patient's arm:**

Gracilis free flap
replacing biceps
muscle defect
and covering
exposed bone

■ Artery
■ Vein
■ Nerve

Figure 3.2 Injury to Konnor's arm with the stages of reconstruction using an innervated gracilis free flap.

Left – an external fixator has been placed to stabilize and reduce the fractured humerus. Center – the gracilis free flap has been sewn into the nearby brachial artery and vein and musculocutaneous nerve. Right – the gracilis free flap replaces the missing biceps muscle.

There were intact, indicating that the radial artery was either in spasm or was being occluded by a distal clot within the lumen. A small bolus of tissue plasminogen activator (TPA) was injected into the radial artery. TPA is a protein that acts as an enzyme and is normally found on endothelial cells, the cells that line blood vessels. It catalyzes the conversion of plasminogen to plasmin, the main enzyme that is responsible for clot breakdown. TPA is routinely used to treat the blood clots that can be responsible for heart attacks, embolic strokes, or pulmonary emboli. The hand became pink; the tissue of the forearm and the wound began to bleed more robustly. With the arm now reliably perfused, the patient was taken to the ICU to continue his resuscitation.

After a crush injury, especially one that has an initial compromised circulation, the soft tissue in the zone of the injury will have some degree of progressive necrosis. Serial exams under anesthesia are done to clean the wound and surgically remove any necrotic tissue. When one is confident that the limits of tissue loss have been reached, definitive orthopedic and plastic surgery management begins. Over the next 10 days, Konnor underwent four debridements and washouts of the arm. Additional nonviable biceps and triceps muscle were debrided. The radial nerve, the nerve responsible for elbow extension (i.e., innervation of the triceps) and extension of the wrist and fingers (i.e., motor innervation of the posterior forearm) was intact, but was missing complete soft tissue coverage. The fractured humerus could be clearly seen.

With the necrotic tissue removed, Dr. Jonathan Barnwell, orthopedic trauma surgeon, removed the external fixator and did an open reduction internal fixation (ORIF) of the fractured humerus. With plates now directly on top of the bone (not externally mounted outside the arm as with an external fixator), the hardware needed to be covered with soft tissue in a coordinated and expedited fashion to decrease the risk of infection in the bone. On the following morning, I began the soft tissue reconstruction.

A large piece of the biceps muscle, as well as the overlying fat, fascia, and skin, was missing. The radial nerve was exposed; without coverage, it would dry up. Elbow, wrist, and finger extension would be permanently decreased. The reconstructive plates and screws holding the bones in place would eventually become infected without coverage. To not decrease blood flow to the forearm, any microvascular anastomosis would have to be done above the zone of injury into the brachial artery and vein. The primary superficial veins of the arm, the cephalic and basilic, as well as the deep veins of the arm accompanying the radial and ulnar artery, were either clotted or likely damaged by the trauma.

The plan for any reconstruction proceeds from an examination of the missing and damaged anatomy, to a determination of what parts of the body have not been damaged (i.e., can be used for harvesting a free flap), to a selection of which vessels into which one can sew. Sew into a damaged vessel, and it will likely clot. Choose a flap with a short pedicle, and the soft tissue of the flap may not fully cover the wound. Do not harvest an anterolateral thigh free flap from a thigh with an underlying femur fracture. Should the flap be a gracilis muscle with a relatively small volume compared to a latissimus muscle with much larger volume? What other fasciocutaneous or musculocutaneous flaps, from the arms, legs, back, or abdomen, could be used so that a skin graft would not be needed to cover a muscle flap? Would these flaps be too heavy and thick because the patient is obese? These general considerations and questions are the initial parameters that guide the surgeon.

"Just get the flap to live" is an imperative that dominates the decisions of relatively inexperienced microsurgeons. Unlike other surgeries, the outcomes of microvascular surgery are without gray. They are black and white. The flap is dead or alive. The patient either needs more surgery, needs an amputation, or does not because the flap has been well designed and technically executed. Beware of the surgeon who blames the patient for a flap failure. Failure can be the result of poor planning or execution. Once flap survival has become an expected outcome in the surgeon's mind, emphasis expands to refinements of function. How can a flap be designed to improve any loss of function associated with the trauma? Can the flap provide more than just soft tissue coverage?

Innervated free muscle flaps have the unique potential of providing not only soft tissue coverage but also muscle contraction. In particular, the gracilis muscle can be harvested with its motor nerve, the obturator nerve, that makes it contact. At the time of the flap transfer, if the obturator nerve is then connected to a nearby motor nerve, the gracilis muscle can contract and also maintain its bulk. Without reconnecting its nerve supply, a muscle flap over time will atrophy, like a muscle that never is used or exercised. For the majority of wounds that simply need soft tissue coverage, the surgeon wants the free muscle to atrophy over time. Otherwise, once the wound and muscle flap have healed, the resulting reconstruction appears too bulky with too much volume.

Patients with facial paralysis present a unique challenge to the microsurgeon and an opportunity to learn how best to perform the transfer of innervated muscle flaps. For a patient who has a complete, long-standing flaccid paralysis either from trauma, tumor surgery, or a congenital anomaly, facial movement can be regained with the transfer of an innervated gracilis muscle (see Figure 2.3). However, how normal the resultant facial movement appears depends on multiple factors. The importance of these factors, not only for facial reanimation but also for improving their use in the reconstruction of an extremity, was underscored by the comments of a previous patient.

Twenty-two months after having had her acoustic neuroma tumor resected, I met Mrs. Nancy M in my biweekly clinic that was focused on seeing patients with facial paralysis. An acoustic neuroma is a benign tumor that develops on the vestibulocochlear nerve leading from the inner ear to the brain. Because the vestibulocochlear neve is next to the facial nerve within the brain, as the tumor grows or as a result of treatment, the facial nerve can become paralyzed, either temporarily or permanently. Mrs. M had severe facial dysfunction. With maximum effort to produce a smile, only the corner of her mouth moved slightly. There was no movement of her forehead, incomplete eye closure, and the corner of her mouth was drooped. By placing a gracilis muscle in her cheek under the skin, I knew I could restore some movement in her midface.

The operation began with an incision similar to a facelift: just below the temporal sideburn, in front of the ear, and then curved slightly into the neck. The skin was lifted up until the corner of the mouth was reached. Just over the body of the mandible in the lower cheek, one can feel the pulses of the facial artery as it heads toward the lip. At this spot in the cheek, one can dissect out the facial artery and vein so that they can be isolated for anastomoses for a gracilis free flap. Underneath the zygomatic arch, the masseter nerve was isolated in order to be the motor nerve that would be sewn to the obturator nerve.

Was the operation a success? The muscle was placed in the cheek; the vessels and nerves were reconnected with restoration of perfusion and neural connection. Then we waited for the nerve to grow, for the transferred muscle to begin contracting.

Three months after surgery, Mrs. M's gracilis muscle began to move. Because the masseter nerve is the normal innervation to a chewing muscle (i.e., the masseter muscle), the patient must at first consciously "bite" to activate the gracilis muscle. Overtime, this activation often becomes more spontaneous so that a patient does not consciously need to "bite" to smile. "That does not look normal, and why does my face appear too full" were the comments of Mrs. M. I reassured her that this would get better over the next few months. At 6 months, the contractions had become stronger. However, the lifting of the corner of the mouth did not match the opposite face. It was too horizontal, and still with a weaker excursion compared to the non-paralyzed side. Moreover, the excessive bulk in the face remained.

As an attending surgeon, the opportunities for learning from your mistakes are much less structured than for a surgeon in training. As an attending, when you question your own results or when a new procedure is introduced, you start by reading what has been published. Perhaps you take a course, typically offered at one of your national annual meetings, or you travel to visit and watch another surgeon do the procedure. Video clips may be available for you to review. I traveled to Toronto to watch Dr. Ronald Zuker, one of the most experienced facial paralysis surgeons at the time, do a similar operation at The Hospital for Sick Children. What was Dr. Zuker doing differently that I should know?

The sewing of the vessels and the nerves was not the focus of the operation. These were taken for granted. What mattered were the fine details, the things that one appreciates only through years of practice and experience. The branching pattern of the obturator nerve into the gracilis muscle was carefully mapped so that the smallest amount of well-innervated muscle would be harvested. Normal fat in the face, buccal fat, was removed so that the bulk introduced by the gracilis would not appear excessive. The vector of the smile on the normal side of the face, the nonparalyzed side, was marked on the skin so that this line of contraction could be exactly matched by placing the gracilis in a similar vector. Before harvesting the gracilis, the length of the muscle was marked in centimeters with a surgical pen so that an exact resting length of muscle could be harvested.

The natural resting length of our skeletal muscles maximizes the ability of the muscle to contract when stimulated. If the resting length is longer or shorter than normal, then the force of contraction decreases. This relationship of the force of contraction to resting length is referred to as the length-tension relationship. In my own research I had raised the hypothesis that if you support partially paralyzed facial muscles with strips of facia that restore the length of the muscle back to a closer, normal resting length, then the force of the smile would increase. Using EMG data, questionnaires, and video analysis, we published our results showing the improved results.[6] Thus, the issue of the importance of the length-tension relationship for optimizing muscle contraction was current in my mind as I watched Dr. Zuker mark the resting length of the gracilis muscle. I could not have imagined that nearly 20 years later, I was going to take this concept of length-tension in facial paralysis to my patient with his arm nearly detached.

"He wanted to be doctor, maybe even a surgeon", Konnor's mom confided to me and the ICU nurse. At 6-foot-2, it was obvious that Konnor was a gifted athlete. At 16 years of age, his physical identity, and his family's peace and security, had irrevocably changed, but there was no self-pity, or at least Konnor did not show it. During his initial evaluation, he had an incidental finding of testing positive for asymptomatic COVID, and then developed an intestinal bacterial infection called C. diff. (*Clostridioide difficile*), with abdominal cramping and watery diarrhea as often as 6 to 10 times a day. Christa Carver, RN, a surgical trauma nurse and friend of the family, commented,

> So here we were, turning this poor (football player sized) teenage boy with external fixation on his right arm and right leg and various fractures, completely onto his side to clean him up multiple times a day/night. He had to be in terrible pain, but he was never rude and he always thanked us after we were done.[7]

"Thank you" was the refrain after each bed turning, meal delivery, and exam during morning rounds. Konnor was polite to everyone regardless of their position. He seemed to want to cheer us up as we discussed the realities of his injuries. The ultimate function of the arm was impossible to predict, but it was not going to be normal.

Speaking to Konnor, I had difficulty not visualizing the image of Bob Dole, holding a pen in his disabled right arm.[8] Senator Dole, former Republican presidential candidate and US Senate Majority Leader, had been a student-athlete on the University of Kansas's football, basketball, and track teams. He had dreamed of becoming a doctor before he enlisted, before he was hit by shrapnel while serving in Italy in World War II. In his 2005 memoir, *One Soldier's Story*, Dole wrote,

> as is often the case with any traumatic blow to a person's physical or emotional well-being, I didn't totally understand the seriousness of my injuries, and I was not ready to accept the fact that my life would be changed forever. On the morning of April 14, 1945, I could raise my right hand high in the air and motion the men in my platoon to follow me. It's been more than sixty years since that morning, and I've not raised my right hand over my head since.
>
> (Dole, p. 160)

The pen served two purposes – it discouraged people in a subtle gesture from shaking his hand, and it was an encouragement. It was his ability that counted, not his disability.

"My greatest fear was that I'd be languishing in a wheelchair, selling pencils on street corners, scrounging to support myself" (Dole, p. 218). In 1996 in a *Time* magazine interview, Dole reflected on the importance of President Franklin D. Roosevelt visibly using his wheelchair during a visit to a military hospital in Hawaii. "He toured the amputee wards in his wheelchair," Dole said. "He went by each bed, letting the men see him exactly as he was. He did not need to give any pep talk – his example said it all".[9]

In 1947, Dole traveled to Chicago to consult with Dr. Hampar Kelikian, one of the top orthopedic surgeons in the country at that time. From a strictly medical point of view, the seven operations that were subsequently performed were less than successful. Little additional function was restored to the arm. Instead, Dr. Kelikian performed a different kind of miracle:

> Dr K was the first doctor to really shoot straight with me. There was something about his transparent honesty, his demeanor, his frank assessment of the situation that caused me to accept his diagnosis – not just of my arms, shoulder, and hands, but of my life … He inspired within me a new attitude, a new way of looking at my life, urging me to focus on what I had left and what I could do with it, rather than complaining about what had been lost and could never be repaired.
>
> (Dole, p. 244)

In later years, through example and legislation, that inspiration blossomed to affect countless persons with disabilities. In 1983 Dole created the Dole Foundation to support programs for those with disabilities. In 1990 he was instrumental in securing passage of the Americans with Disabilities Act. The Americans with Disabilities Act ensured local and state government facilities and services, as well as private employers, could no longer discriminate against individuals with disabilities. "He as a person with a disability, knowing his own potential and the desire to be an independent and fully participatory individual and in the economy and in our society – that's what he wanted this legislation to do," said Audrey Coleman, director of the Robert J. Dole Institute of Politics at the University of Kansas.[10]

The potential of Konnor's arm, including the possibility of even keeping the arm, was now my responsibility. Trauma and orthopedic surgery were done. The arm was perfused; the remaining tissue was healthy; the humerus was now in its proper position. However, the arm was naked without skin; the plates, the nerves, and the gap in the muscles were all fully exposed (Figure 3.2). Between the septum separating the biceps brachii and the brachialis (the two main flexors of the elbow), there it was – the musculocutaneous nerve. This nerve is the main motor nerve to the biceps brachii and the brachialis. The brachialis was partially torn but relatively intact, and importantly, I could see branches of the musculocutaneous nerve entering the brachialis deep to the missing biceps brachii.

Could I design an innervated muscle free flap? Maybe – I would have to sew into the brachial artery and vein above the zone of injury. Dissected out, these vessels were now 6 cm above the gap in the muscle. Put the arm at full elbow extension to measure the resting length of the missing biceps brachii. Now the muscle defect measured 7 cm in length and 5 cm in width. I still needed a motor nerve in the arm to which I could sew the transplanted nerve from the free muscle flap. I should not divide any of the remaining branches from the musculocutaneous nerve to the brachialis, because this would decrease the remaining elbow flexion. By the dissected brachial artery and vein, I isolated the larger trunk of the musculocutaneous nerve for a possible end to side neurorrhaphy.

In peripheral nerve surgery, an end-to-side neurorrhaphy involves sewing the end of one nerve into the side of the trunk of an adjacent nerve. Experimental and clinical data have shown that an end-to-side neurorrhaphy can provide innervation into the recipient nerve without causing a decrease in the function of the muscle(s) that are supplied by the main trunk of the donor nerve. The accepted mechanism is that collateral nerves sprout from the main trunk from the small window that is made in the side of the nerve and then grow into the recipient nerve.

A 15-centimeter incision was made in the skin of the left medial thigh. The glistening fat sprang out. The greater saphenous vein poked into the field and was retracted out of the way. The white, thin fascia wrapping the gracilis muscle was carefully divided with a scalpel. Now the real finesse of the operation began. The muscle was rolled medially to isolate the obturator nerve innervating the gracilis muscle and to identify the entry point of the vascular pedicle into the muscle. With the muscle not yet cut, centimeter marks were drawn on the muscle. For contraction to be its maximum, the length of the transplanted gracilis had to equal exactly the 7 cm resting gap of the biceps. One centimeter would be added on each end of the muscle to account for the bunching of the gracilis caused by sewing the muscle into place. The vascular pedicle was dissected back to the profundus artery, the main deep arterial and venous supply of the thigh. The vascular pedicle was 7 cm in length with an artery that measured 1.5 mm in diameter and with two veins, each about 2.5 mm. These vessels would be sewn with end-to-side anastomoses into the brachial artery and vein. The gracilis artery and veins would have to be dissected from each other, separated for about 2 cm, to obtain adequate length and freedom of movement to make the anastomoses technically easier.

Vessel loops were placed around the brachial artery and vein. The operating microscope was positioned over the brachial vessels in the arm and adjusted to an 8x magnification. The divided muscle, now on ischemia time, was first sewn into the cut end of the distal biceps muscle. The vessel loops were tightened to stop blood flow to the arm, and with a pointed knife, a number 11 scalpel, I sliced a tiny hole into the brachial artery. Fine 8.0 suture, the size of a human hair, was then used to sew the gracilis artery into the brachial artery. A similar anastomosis was done for one of the gracilis veins to the brachial vein. The vessel loops were relaxed, and instantly the hand became pink, as well as the gracilis flap.

Now focus on innervation. The flap is alive but will not contract without the nerve. Like tapping a maple tree for syrup, make sure the hole is not too large or deep to cause injury. Visualizing the white trunk of the musculocutaneous nerve with 8x magnification, the outer layer of the nerve, the epineurium, was incised to allow visualization of the underlying nerve fascicles. The cable-like bundle of white glistening fascicles bulged through the small window. Then three 8.0 sutures were used to sew the epineurium of the obturator nerve to the edges cut into the epineurium of the musculocutaneous nerve. Only now could the muscle be fully laid across the defect in the biceps and brought out to length; otherwise, the muscle would have obstructed the view of underlying brachial vessels and musculocutaneous nerve (see Figure 3.2).

Like Bob Dole, Konnor was also a Boy Scout. A Boy Scout lives by 12 principles, which are considered the Scout Law: "A scout is trustworthy, loyal, helpful, friendly, courteous, kind, obedient, cheerful, thrifty, brave, clean, and reverent". During the years before the accident, Konnor had been on the path of becoming an Eagle Scout. Only about 5% of scouts go on to become Eagle Scouts. What is special about Eagle Scouts is grit. To achieve the rank, you must set on the path at an early age. They set goals and have the persistence and discipline to achieve these goals. Twenty-one merit badges, focused on acquiring skills that contribute to society as a whole, are required before you turn 18 years of age.

"When can I start using my arm?" was nearly the first question that Konnor asked after surgery. Ten days after his gracilis free flap, Konnor was discharged from the hospital, and within a few weeks he began physical therapy to improve the strength and range of movement of his right arm.

With the grit of an Eagle Scout, Konnor has made remarkable progress. Christa Carver, a family friend, wrote:

> In the last 11 months, Konnor has absolutely crushed physical therapy, going above and beyond every challenge posed to him. Not only has he returned to school on his feet, he has more use of his right arm and hand than anyone imagined he could! He has completed his Eagle Scout and lit the candle at his ceremony (with his right hand)!! [Figure 3.3] He was the football team manager for his high school this fall. He will graduate from high school this spring and has already decided to study pre-med, and it seems he will have his choice of several programs. ... He hopes to be able to help trauma patients in their recovery of function.[11]

Just 6 months later, the family updated Konnor's progress with a note to the trauma team:

> Konnor graduated from high school last week and will be going to Alaska in a couple of weeks. He'll have then visited all 50 states, which was his Dad's goal for the family. He has been accepted to CU [Colorado University] in Denver and plans to study biology with the goal of further education for a career in Orthopedic Surgery.[12]

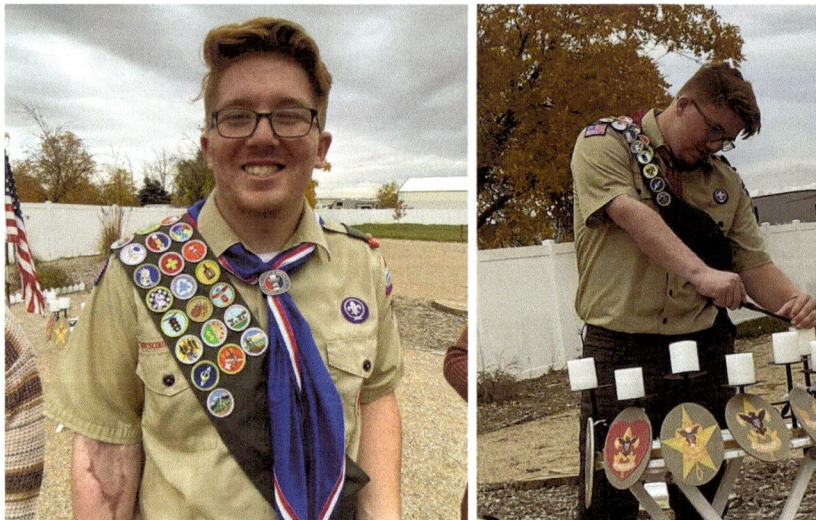

Figure 3.3 Konnor earning his Eagle Scout rank and using his reconstructed arm to light the ceremonial candle.

Courtesy of Konnor Burge.

Konnor, from the many doctors and nurses who had the privilege to care for you, thank you. Why we submerge ourselves so completely in taking care of patients has been justified.

A total life adjustment is not uncommon after a disability. Fortunately, people have a capacity for adjustment after a catastrophic injury. We optimize our strengths and learn to compensate for the areas in which we struggle. However, pain control can be an insurmountable problem for many patients with limb trauma. At an amputation site and even in a salvaged limb, pain can be relentless, burning, shooting. The agony can make a patient feel hopeless, angry, desperate. "Your state of life is a reflection of your state of mind." If pain cannot be controlled, it will destroy a person.

"Please I do not want a lot of pain pills. I have some friends who have had problems with oxycontin!" These were nearly the first words that Mr. Steve B voiced when I met him awake for the first time. Two days prior, having just lifted a crate onto a shelf in the distribution center, Steve turned to walk around the forklift behind him. The crush of the forklift into his left leg as it pushed and trapped him against a pillar was his last memory as he faded from blood loss and pain. In the trauma bay of the emergency department, the tourniquet on the thigh was gently released. An instant gush of blood spilled onto the bed. A gaping hole traversed the thigh. There was no pulse below the knee; the quadriceps and femur were exploded.

Whisked to the operating room, the trauma surgeons cut through the medial thigh to obtain access to the femoral artery just above the knee. Vessel loops were passed around the artery and vein and pulled up. With blood flow now stopped, the damage could be assessed. The popliteal artery and vein, the main and only blood supply, to the lower leg were transected just behind the knee. The remaining anatomy was unrecognizable. The calf and thigh muscles were fragmented, missing, and ripped from their points of insertion on the tibia and femur. The main motor and sensory nerve extending from the thigh into the calf (i.e., the distal sciatic nerve) was in pieces, missing at the site of impalement. Pieces of the femur were floating in the wound. Could this leg be salvaged? Should this leg be salvaged?

It is an unfair question. Would you acutely amputate a leg if you knew that technically you could reconnect it, but the patient may be left with chronic pain and dysfunction?

"Doc, just cut it off". There is the rare patient who tells you before a reconstructive effort that he has had enough. Mr. F was such a patient. He was an active 45-year-old biker with arms and a chest ripped from years of being a bodybuilder. From his motorcycle crash, his distal tibia and ankle were fractured in multiple pieces, with the skin and soft tissue missing over the fractures. The fractures had been reduced with an external fixator, and a VAC (i.e., Vacuum-Assisted Closure) sponge had been placed over the open wound as a dressing. At the bedside, the attending orthopedic surgeon and I outlined the subsequent operations and risks that would be needed to salvage the leg. The external fixator would be removed, and the fractures would be plated internally. The wound would then be covered with a free flap also on that day. After the flap had healed, the patient would need additional surgery in the following few months to provide bone grafts to augment and replace the missing bone. The ankle may need to be fused. During these months as he healed, the patient would not be able to bear weight on the leg. The bone could become infected; the flap could clot; he may have chronic pain. "I cannot sit around and do all of that. Cut it off!", was Mr. F's response.

There was no possible conversation to be had with Mr. B. He was intubated on the operating table. We made the emergent decision to try to salvage the leg. With the popliteal transection recognized, vascular surgery went to work. The right leg was scanned with ultrasound for a long enough vein to be harvested so that a bypass graft could be sewn around the popliteal transection. The veins were either not long enough or were damaged. The nurse circulator rushed to the storage room and retrieved a cadaveric saphenous vein graft from the shelf. It was not from the patient. However, it still could work, even though it had a slightly higher rate of clotting compared to an autologous vein. The vascular surgeon cut around the ankle to isolate the distal posterior tibial artery, well away from the site of the trauma. Above the popliteal artery, a slit was cut into the superficial femoral artery (SFA). Blood shot out as the clot was extracted with a catheter. Then a long tunnel was made just underneath the intact skin of the calf down to the ankle. One last check was done to be sure the graft was not twisted as it was passed through the tunnel. Nimbly, the vascular surgeon sewed the graft into the SFA and posterior tibial artery. Clamps were released (Figure 3.4).

Circulation was restored to the leg, but for how long? The vein graft was strung across a void of missing tissue where the thigh musculature should have been. Without soft tissue coverage around the graft, it was just a matter of time until it clotted or burst. "I cannot feel that," was Mr. B's response the next day as we poked his foot with a needle. "I want to keep my leg. Do whatever you think is necessary. I understand that it may not work after the operation." So, 2 days after the accident, I harvested a lattisimus free flap from the patient's chest. The vessels of the flap were sewn end-to-side in the SFA and SFV above the site of the vein graft. Through the hole the size of my fist, the latissimus flap was wrapped around the vein graft, around the fractured femur, and then passed to the lateral aspect of the knee where the flap was turned over on itself to cover the knee where skin was missing.

Over the next 10 days four additional major operations were needed. Four days after the flap, the external fixator was replaced with an internal rod that was placed through the fractured femur. During the manipulation of the leg, the vein graft clotted. The vascular surgeon and I reopened the leg, pulled out the clot, and repaired the partially torn vein. Heparin, a powerful blood thinner, was started as a continuous drip through an intravenous line to prevent more clots. It did its job too well. Other vessels in the leg began to bleed, and the patient returned emergently to the operating room

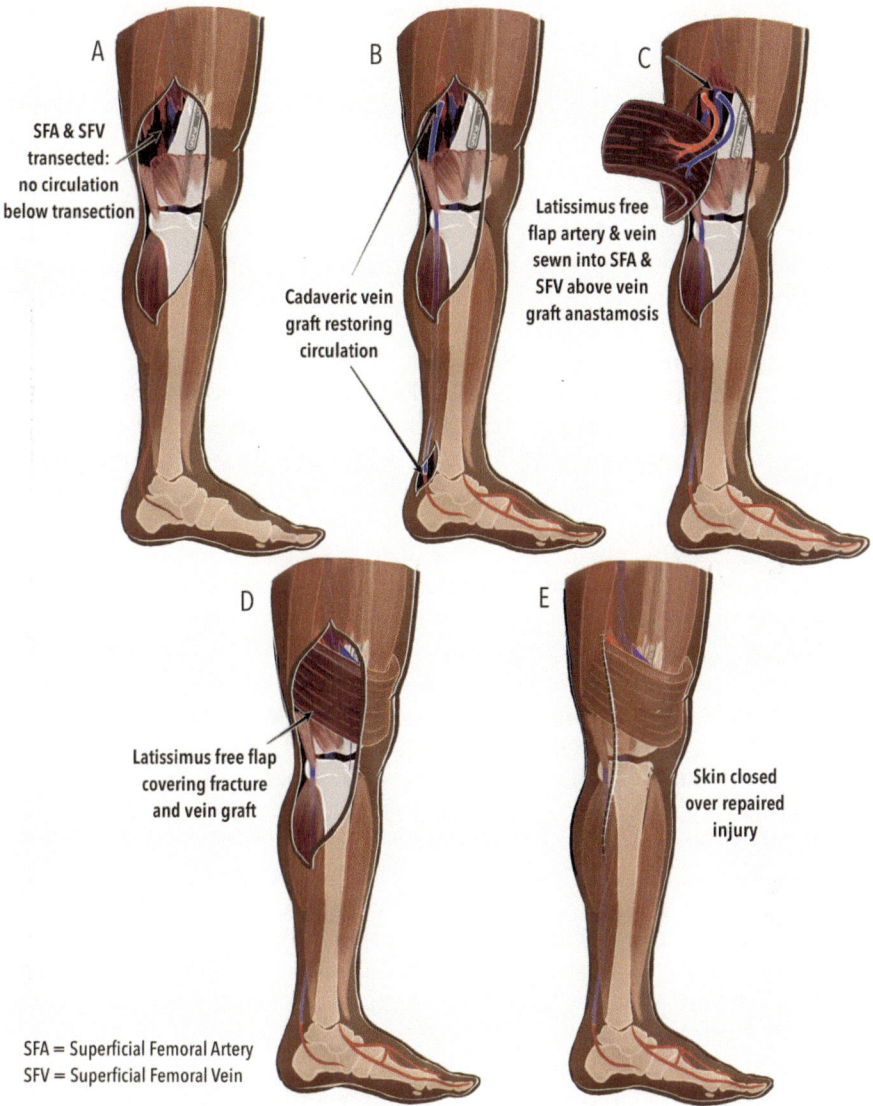

A

SFA & SFV
transected:
no circulation
below transection

B

Cadaveric vein
graft restoring
circulation

C

Latissimus free
flap artery & vein
sewn into SFA &
SFV above vein
graft anastamosis

D

Latissimus free flap
covering fracture
and vein graft

E

Skin closed
over repaired
injury

SFA = Superficial Femoral Artery
SFV = Superficial Femoral Vein

Figure 3.4 Lower extremity salvage with restoration of perfusion with vein graft
and coverage with a latissimus free flap.

**The main artery to the leg has been transected. A vein graft has been
used to bypass the transection to restore circulation below the knee
(second panel). A lattisimus free flap has been sewn into the circulation
above the transection and then draped over the zone of injury to protect the vein graft and to cover the fractured femur.**

so that these could be cauterized and ligated. The heparin was stopped. Skin grafts to cover the exposed latissimus muscle was the final stage, done 10 days after the flap.

The electric shocks shooting through the extremity began as early as 4 days after the injury. Though maybe sooner, before that time Mr. B was still regaining clarity of thought, as he awoke from the effects of the anesthetics and narcotics. "The pain does not let me think. It is currently a 9 out 10 and is most often a 10/10. It never goes below an 8/10." Acute pain right after an injury or a surgery is considered a protective nociceptive response. Nociceptors, special nerve cells, send warning signals (i.e., pain) along the peripheral nerves back to the brain. It is the normal response when somatic structures such as skin, muscle, tendon, or bone are injured. Neuropathic pain is a different type of pain. It is linked to damage of the body's neurological system. The incidence increases after major nerve injury or transections with an estimated prevalence of 50%–80% in patients who have undergone an amputation. It is typically referred to as nerve pain and persists after the wounds have healed and inflammation has subsided. It can be chronic and life-altering.

In the last few decades there has been a paradigm shift in the management of pain for surgical patients, especially those who have suffered major unexpected trauma. This shift has focused on multimodal pain control with limited opioid use, and the prompt utilization of behavior health and psychiatry.[13] New persistent opioid use is a common postoperative complication, with 6% of previously opioid-naïve patients continuing to fill opioid prescriptions 3–6 months after surgery. This risk increases to about 20% in opioid-naïve patients undergoing a major amputation. Gabapentoids, antidepressants, acetaminophen, nonsteroidal anti-inflammatory medications (i.e., ibuprofen), local anesthetics, and regional nerve blocks have the potential to reduce the severity of acute and chronic pain. In a systematic and timely manner, the combination of Steve's medications was started, increased, and adjusted.

However, what seemed to matter the most were the coping skills and interventions introduced by the behavioral health team. Nearly every day, Laura or Brandy (the names have been changed), two of the dedicated behavior health counselors, would focus on breathing exercises and other cognitive skills to help Steve with his anxiety and depression. Laura commented, "Steve is quite stoic, fights against showing tears as we discuss the injury and what life may look like after discharge." "Please come back tomorrow and check on me. I like to be able to talk with people" was a daily sentiment. This simple daily human contact was what seemed to help Steve the most in coping with his pain.

Bob Dole expressed a similar revelation in his book:

> To visit soldiers who have been injured, or anyone who is dealing with a disability that confines him or her to a hospital bed can be emotionally draining. But it's hard to overestimate how important and meaningful

such visits can be. Some people avoid visiting someone who is incapacitated because they worry that they won't know what to say. Truth is you probably don't need to say much of anything. You can be a tremendous encouragement to someone just by being there.

(Dole, p. 161)

Five weeks after the accident, Steve was discharged from the hospital to live with his sister. His treating psychiatrist succinctly summarized: "the pain is tolerable, and the patient is future oriented". Steve is still at great risk for addiction, because he is likely to be left with chronic pain. His chronic narcotic use is being managed by a pain specialist. Antidepressant medications and cognitive therapy are ongoing. His leg is attached. However, the limb salvage was not simply a surgery. It is now a lifelong commitment between Steve, the multiple medical teams that are still caring for him, and, hopefully, the people closest to him.

REFERENCES

1. NIH, US National Library of Medicine. *Maimed Men – Life and Limb: The Toll of the American Civil War*, March 17, 2011 (https://www.nlm.nih.gov/exhibition/lifeandlimb/maimedmen.html).
2. Office of the Surgeon General, Department of the Army. *The Medical Department of the United States Army in World War II*, 1970 Jan:304–305.
3. Baker MS. Lead, follow, or get out of the way – how bold young surgeons brought vascular surgery into clinical practice from the Korean War battlefield. *Ann Vasc Surg* 2016;33:258–262.
4. Shoeib MA. Cross-leg flap: Its reliability and outcome. *Modern Plastic Surgery*, 2013;3:9–14.
5. UCHealth writers. Young man thanks Memorial trauma team for saving his life. October 31, 2022 (https://bit.ly/UCHealthYouTube).
6. Deleyiannis FWB, Askari M, Schmidt KL, Henkelmann TC, VanSwearingen JM, Mander EK. Muscle activity in the partially paralyzed face after placement of a fascial sling: a preliminary report. *Ann Plast Surg*. 2005 Nov;55(5):449–455.
7. Carver C., personal correspondence, January 2021.
8. Bob Dole. *One Soldier's Story: A Memoir*. HarperCollins Publishers, 2005.
9. Ducharme J. Bob Dole lived with a disability for decades: Here's how it shaped his life and legacy. *Time*, December 5, 2021 (https://www.time.com/How-Bob-Dole's-Life-and-Legacy-Was-Shaped-by-Disability).
10. Taborda N. Bob Dole championed "lives of greater dignity" for Americans with disabilities. *Kansas Reflector*, December 6, 2021 (https://kansasreflector.com).
11. Carver C., email, November 24, 2021.
12. Communications from Burge family, email, June 3, 2022.
13. Urits I, Hubble A, Peterson E, Orhurhu V, Ernst CA, Kaye AD, Viswanath O. An update on cognitive therapy for the management of chronic pain: a comprehensive review. *Curr Pain Headache Rep*. 2019 Jul 10;23(8):57.

Chapter 4

Breast reconstruction

Technical ease, money, and disparity

Everyone should have enough money to get Plastic Surgery.
— Beverly Johnson (American model, 1959–present)

"We want a flap; tell us about it!" In a plastic surgery consultation, especially in the discussion of multiple surgical options, there are two extremes on how patients involve themselves in the decision making. On one end there is the patient who simply states, "Doc, do what you think is best." At the other extreme is the patient who knows everything about you and is prepared to ask everything. They know where you went to medical school, how many articles you have published, have actually read some of these articles, and are ready to tell you their opinion of the best treatment approach. Their opinion is usually right.

Lydia and Kurt Friese were right in their decision about breast reconstruction. It is a tough decision. "I want to go all natural" was the principle guiding Lydia. For women with breast cancer post-mastectomy reconstruction can be done either with breast implants or with your own tissue, usually either from your abdomen or back (i.e., referred to as autologous reconstruction).

Autologous reconstruction has several advantages compared to breast implants. The obvious advantage is the absence of a foreign body with the potential of feeling and looking more natural. In addition to restoring volume, autologous reconstruction (i.e., a flap) can reconstruct a skin defect of the breast (for example, when the nipple is removed), making virtually all mastectomy defects amenable to reconstruction. However, there are disadvantages. The surgery is usually longer and technically more demanding, especially with free flaps. Donor site morbidity, such as pain and wound breakdown at the harvest site, can occur. Depending on the defect, the main flaps used for autologous reconstruction are a pedicled latissimus dorsi flap with an implant, or an abdomen-based flap, such as a deep inferior epigastric artery perforator (DIEP) flap or a pedicled TRAM (transverse rectus abdominis myocutaneous) flap.[1,2]

A pedicled TRAM flap involves using the abdominal skin, fat, and rectus abdominis muscle and rotating it from the lower abdomen into the

 DOI: 10.1201/9781003538028-5

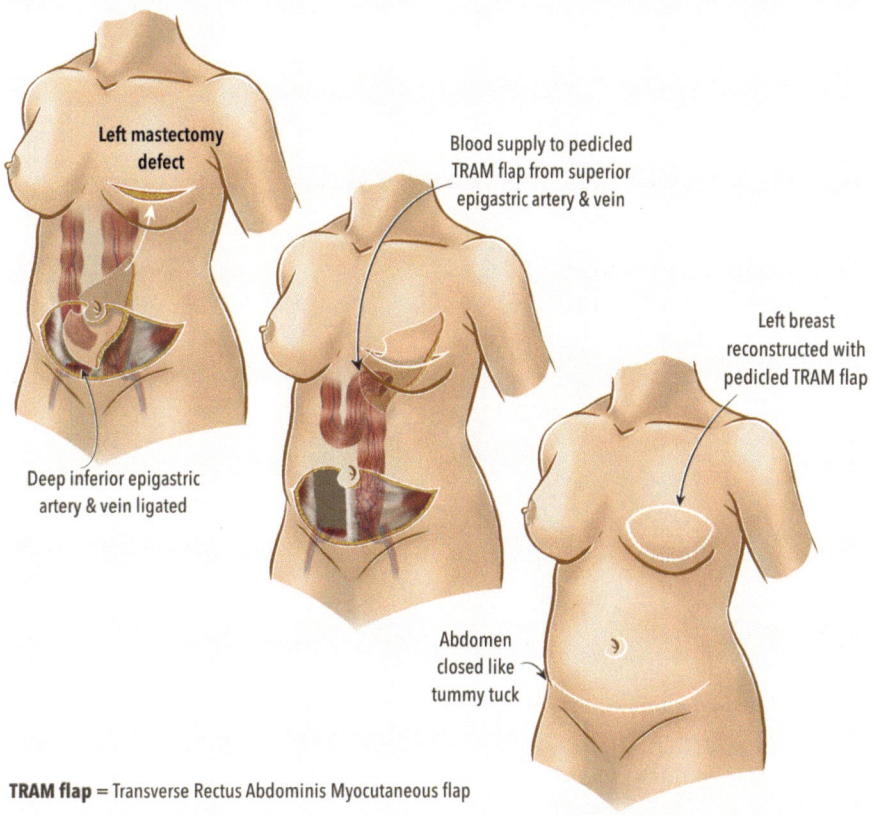

Left mastectomy defect

Blood supply to pedicled TRAM flap from superior epigastric artery & vein

Left breast reconstructed with pedicled TRAM flap

Deep inferior epigastric artery & vein ligated

Abdomen closed like tummy tuck

TRAM flap = Transverse Rectus Abdominis Myocutaneous flap

Figure 4.1 Pedicled transverse rectus abdominis myocutaneous (TRAM) flap.

For a pedicled TRAM flap, microsurgery is not needed, but a large portion of the rectus abdominis muscle is harvested.

mastectomy site (Figure 4.1). The blood vessels of the transferred flap remain attached, as the flap is tunneled under the skin of the upper abdomen. Weakness and hernia of the abdominal wall can occur with abdomen-based flaps, but these have become less of a concern with the evolution of perforator flaps, such as the DIEP flap. With DIEP flaps, less, if any, muscle or fascia is harvested, thus maintaining the integrity of the abdominal wall. The deep inferior epigastric artery (i.e., DIEA), the main arterial blood supply to a DIEP flap, is also more robust than the superior epigastric artery, the main blood supply to a superiorly, pedicled TRAM flap (Figure 4.2). Other free flaps, from the buttocks or thighs, can also be used for breast reconstruction, but these are mainly reserved for patients who are too thin for an abdomen-based free flap or have undergone a pervious tummy tuck (i.e., abdominoplasty).

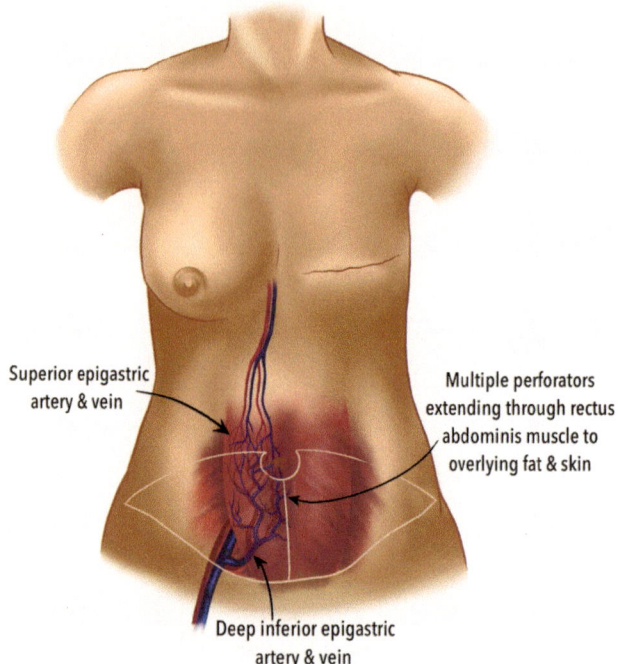

Superior epigastric
artery & vein

Multiple perforators
extending through rectus
abdominis muscle to
overlying fat & skin

Deep inferior epigastric
artery & vein

Figure 4.2 Blood supply to the lower abdominal wall.

The deep inferior epigastric artery (i.e., DIEA) and superior epigastric artery travel underneath and through the rectus abdominis muscle to supply the overlying fat and skin. The DIEA is larger providing greater and more reliable perfusion.

Vast variations exist in the reconstructive options that breast cancer patients are offered. Navigating these options with a patient begins with presenting the average outcomes based on the specific treatment and then layering in how these outcomes may change based on multiple patient factors. In particular, how could the surgical outcome improve or worsen based on the characteristics of the specific patient sitting in front of you? How large and ptotic the patient's breasts are, whether the patient is obese, whether radiation therapy will be needed, and what other illnesses or surgeries the patient has had in the past are the typical questions one considers. Does the patient already have a preference about reconstruction with an implant or with tissue from their own body?

Thanks to the Women's Health and Cancer Rights Act in 1998, all insurance carriers are required to cover breast reconstruction, as well as procedures on the non-cancer breast to create breast symmetry. Implant/tissue expander reconstruction is the most common type of reconstruction preformed in the United States. According to the 2022 data of the American

Society of Plastic Surgery (ASPS), 151,641 operations for breast reconstruction were done annually. Of these, only 14.6% were respectively performed with DIEP flaps (19,857) or free TRAM flaps (2,223), whereas 77.8% were reconstructed either with a tissue expander and implant (82,597) or directly with a breast implant (35,360).[3]

Implant reconstruction, especially in nipple-sparing mastectomies in small-breasted women can have excellent aesthetic results. Such aesthetic results and patient satisfaction typically decrease as breast size increases, the nipple is removed, and/or if radiation therapy is delivered to the mastectomy site/reconstructed breast. Multiple complications can occur with implant-based reconstruction. Implants can feel uncomfortable, become malpositioned, rupture, and/or become infected and need removal. A hard capsule (i.e., capsular contracture) can form around the implant. The risk of these complications increases with obesity, breast ptosis, large breast size, radiation therapy, and other patient factors, such as diabetes and smoking. Re-operation rates have been reported to be as high as 30%–40%, particularly after radiotherapy.

The Mastectomy Reconstruction Outcome Consortium (MROC), a large national multicenter collaboration established in 2012, has extensively studied surgical outcomes of women undergoing breast reconstruction.[4] The consortium included 57 plastic surgeons in 11 centers throughout North America. In an original cohort of 1,632 patients one year after surgery, those who had undergone autologous reconstruction (493 patients) reported greater satisfaction with their breasts and greater psychosocial and sexual well-being compared to those who had undergone implant reconstruction (1,139 patients). Numerous other studies have similarly demonstrated better quality-of-life results comparing autologous reconstruction to implant reconstruction.

The adverse effects of radiation therapy on breast reconstruction, including decreased perfusion to mastectomy flaps, increased capsular contracture around an implant, pain, wound healing complications, and infection, are well known. In a subset analysis of 150 patient enrolled in the MROC study who underwent post-mastectomy radiation therapy and two-stage immediate breast reconstruction with a tissue expander and breast implant, the overall complication rate was 28.7% at one year after mastectomy.[5] Surgical site infection was the highest complication at 14.7% (22 patients). Sixteen (10.7%) women had their implants removed with no additional replacement. At 2-year follow-up, the overall rates of complications and reconstruction failures continued to increase. At 2 years, the total complication rate was now 40.3%. Nearly 20% (17.8%) of the patients had their implants removed. These data are well known to breast surgeons and plastic surgeons. However, each year a growing number of women who will receive radiation are choosing or are being guided toward implant reconstruction. Some patients may not be good candidates for autologous reconstruction. Others may say, "No, I don't want a big operation, give me the implants even if they are not natural, and may need to be removed."

Lydia had extraordinary help from her husband, Kurt, to navigate her decision about breast reconstruction. Kurt had been a chiropractor since 1985. In his practice he helped his own patients advance their health. With his wife as his primary patient now, Kurt delved into medical research and journals. When I first met them, the list of questions was long and sophisticated. It was the best type of consult, informed and based on data.

Lydia and Kurt Frieses' journey with breast cancer began more than a year prior to our first consultation.[6] In January 2017, Lydia began to wonder if something was wrong. As weather systems rolled in and dropped snow across the Front Range, her right breast would begin to ache. "It just didn't feel right", Lydia commented. She asked her husband, for whom touch was his livelihood, to examine her. "When I felt it, there were 4 little nodules, and they were probably like the half size of a pea". The skin over the mass in the upper inner quadrant of the breast also seemed too thick and wrinkled.

A digital mammogram with tomosynthesis (i.e., a diagnostic 3D mammogram) and a subsequent MRI confirmed the presence of a tumor. It was not confined to just the upper inner quadrant. It was multicentric, involving a second site in the upper outer quadrant of the breast. It did not appear to have spread to the lymph nodes in the armpit (i.e., the axillary lymph nodes). However, these would still need to be checked at the time of the mastectomy. The tumor was too extensive for Lydia to be a good candidate for a lumpectomy. The multidisciplinary breast tumor board met to discuss the case. Dr. S, the breast oncology surgeon, recommended a mastectomy. To minimize the extent of possible nodal surgery in the armpit and to potentially make the resection of the tumor easier, in particular off the underlying pectoralis muscle, medical oncology recommended chemotherapy before surgery. Whether radiation therapy would be needed would be based on the final pathology of the mastectomy specimen and the lymph nodes. Two weeks after the Valentine's Day confirmation of her cancer, Lydia began chemotherapy.

After 2 rounds of chemotherapy, lasting about 5 months, Lydia underwent the planned mastectomy and sentinel lymph node biopsies of the axilla. Decades of research have proven that large breast surgeries are often unnecessary. Women with unifocal DCIS (ductal carcinoma in situ) and small invasive cancers have the same chance of survival whether they have a lumpectomy followed by radiation, or a mastectomy. Some women may choose to have a mastectomy to avoid the radiation treatment recommended with a lumpectomy. In agreement with the theme that less is better, breast surgeons leave nearly all of the mastectomy patient's skin in place, scooping out the breast from its skin envelope. A small ellipse is usually cut around the nipple, allowing resection of the nipple, a small amount of skin, and the breast mound. Called a skin-sparing mastectomy, the resulting space is routinely filled either with a tissue expander, implant, or free flap at the same time as the mastectomy.

Small, well-defined mastectomy defects can often be reconstructed with directly placing an implant (i.e., called direct-to-implant reconstruction). To adjust this space and to potentially put less pressure on the mastectomy skin flaps, surgeons often place tissue expanders at the time of the mastectomy. The expanders contain an internal port through which saline can be injected in several sessions in the office after surgery. The saline causes the expander to become progressively larger, stretching the skin and muscle. Once the desired volume and breast size are reached, the tissue expander is exchanged for a breast implant at a second surgery. If it is uncertain whether a patient will receive radiation therapy, a tissue expander is often the preferred choice. The expander can hold the skin envelope in the shape and size of a breast mound. Once the radiation is complete, the expander can be removed and replaced with autologous tissue, such as a DIEP flap. The DIEP has not been radiated, so it feels and heals like normal tissue.

Dr. S worked with a local plastic surgeon and performed the mastectomy and the immediate breast reconstruction with placement of a tissue expander. Before the surgery began, a radioactive tracer had been injected into Lydia's cancerous breast. The tracer courses through the breast's lymphatic systems and is deposited into the primary lymph nodes in the axillae that drain the breast. These "sentinel" nodes are rendered temporarily radioactive so that they can be easier to find and remove during surgery. Dr. S waved a wand called a gamma probe over the area. The wand, a sort of Geiger counter, beeped more intensely when waved over the nodes that contained the radioactive tracer. Dr. S, working through the same incision for the mastectomy, removed the three lymph nodes with the greatest beep.

The reconstruction then began. The plastic surgeon sewed a piece of acellular dermal matrix (ADM) to the lower border of the pectoralis muscle to create an internal sling for the tissue expander. This cadaveric tissue, ADM, is a piece of skin that is specially processed to remove all cells that could lead to tissue rejection. What is left is a matrix that looks like a thick piece of skin. Into this matrix a patient's own cells can grow. The tissue expander was placed underneath the pectoralis, the ADM was draped over the bottom half of the tissue expander, and the ADM was then sewn to the inframammary breast fold. The skin incision was closed, leaving a transverse line across the site where the nipple had been. Where Lydia's breast had been was now a small breast mound created by the partially inflated tissue expander.

Seven days later Dr. S reviewed the pathology finding with the Frieses. The mastectomy margins were clear. The breast cancer had been completely removed with the mastectomy. However, one of the sentinel lymph nodes had a small collection of cancer cells, and the main cancer within the breast had little to no response to the chemotherapy. Tumor cells could still be found within the breast tissue. Because of the residual cancer within the lymph node and the breast, radiotherapy was recommended. Weighing the options with her radiation oncologist, Lydia chose to enter a clinical study that would be a shorter time frame with higher radiation dosages. Lydia started a 19-day trial 2 weeks before Thanksgiving and completed in on December 12, 2017.

Four months after radiation therapy completion, I met Kurt and Lydia for the first time in consultation. "I told Dr. D what I wanted was the flap and what my husband had explained to me is that it's a tough surgery". Kurt and Lydia already knew the data on poor outcomes for patients with implants and radiation. It would take a number of weeks to heal after the DIEP free flap, but there would be no implant, and importantly, no long-term risk of implant-associated failure. Lydia rightly believed that the DIEP flap would provide her with a more natural-looking breast. "First, it would be my own tissue", she said. "Second, because it was my own tissue, I wouldn't need regular MRIs as follow-ups to check the integrity of an implant over the future decades. ... Finally, as a side benefit, I had a tummy tuck". The radiation therapy made Lydia look as though she had a bad sunburn on the right side of her chest. We would wait an additional 3 months before performing the DIEP surgery to allow the skin to heal from the acute radiation effects.

The day arrived. Lydia checked in about 5:30 a.m., and Kurt was at her side until 7:30 a.m., when she was wheeled into the operating room. The breast skin overlying the now fully expanded tissue expander was still slightly darker but no longer angry. It was tense with little mobility from the scarring caused by the radiation. "Do not worry; we will take good care of you". With this final reassurance, Lydia drifted off to sleep. Her skin from the neck to the mid thighs was prepped with Betadine antiseptic. Dr Nancy Wong, my practice partner, and I began the operation.

Working simultaneously, two surgeons can cut hours off the time necessary for the operation. This is especially true in bilateral breast reconstructions with two DIEPs. Dr. Wong reopened the horizontal incision across the right breast and removed the tissue expander. The cavity was lined with a stiff capsule, like cardboard. A cautery was used to make transverse and longitudinal cuts in the capsule to release it. The standard recipient vessels for a DIEP flap are the artery and vein(s) that lie just below the ribs lateral to the sternum, the internal mammary artery (IMA) and vein (IMV). To expose these vessels, Dr. Wong removed a small section of the overlying third rib (Figure 4.3). Only the parietal pleura, a thin layer of transparent connective tissue, separates these vessels from the underlying lung. The gray sponge of the lung could be seen filling and evacuating with each breath from the ventilator. As every heart surgeon knows, the IMA is the preferred vessel for a cardiac bypass, because it is so close to the heart. Injury to the lung from preparing the IMA and IMV as recipient vessels is an almost unheard-of complication, rare but still possible. However, as part of an informed consent, it is mentioned to the patient.

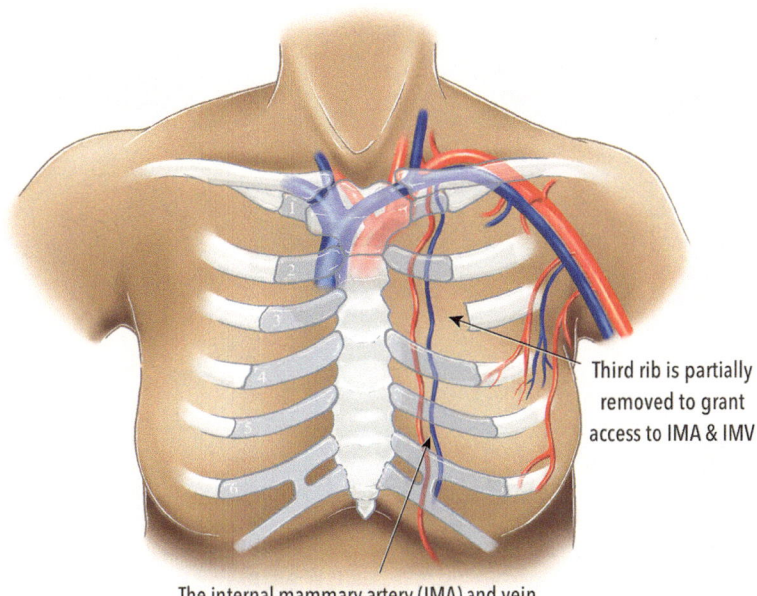

Third rib is partially
removed to grant
access to IMA & IMV

The internal mammary artery (IMA) and vein
(IMV) are typically used as recipient vessels

Figure 4.3 Preparation of the recipient vessels for a deep inferior epigastric perforator (DIEP) free flap.

The recipient vessels for a Deep Inferior Epigastric Perforator (DIEP) Free Flap are typically the Internal Mammary Artery (IMV) and Vein (IMV) located underneath the medial ribs.

While Dr. Wong isolated the IMA and IMV, I began to harvest the DIEP flap (Figure 4.4). The incisions and the tissue removed are essentially the same as those of an abdominoplasty, "a tummy tuck". For a unilateral breast reconstruction, one-half of the lower abdomen is generally used; the other half is discarded. The perforators which supply the skin and fat of the lower abdomen originate from the deep inferior epigastric artery (DIEA) and vein (DIEV), which originate from the external iliac artery and vein in the groin and then run superiorly underneath and into the rectus abdominis muscle (Figure 4.4). The perforators pierce the muscle and the anterior rectus fascia to pass into the fat and the skin. When a tummy tuck is done, these perforators are clipped and cauterized so they do not bleed, and the entire skin and fat from the belly button to the superior pubic area is excised and discarded. For DIEP flap, these perforators must be carefully identified. The largest one or two perforators is then chosen and dissected back through the rectus muscle into the larger DIEA and DIEV. If chosen and dissected properly, the perforators provide a robust blood supply to the harvested abdominal skin and fat that will become the breast.

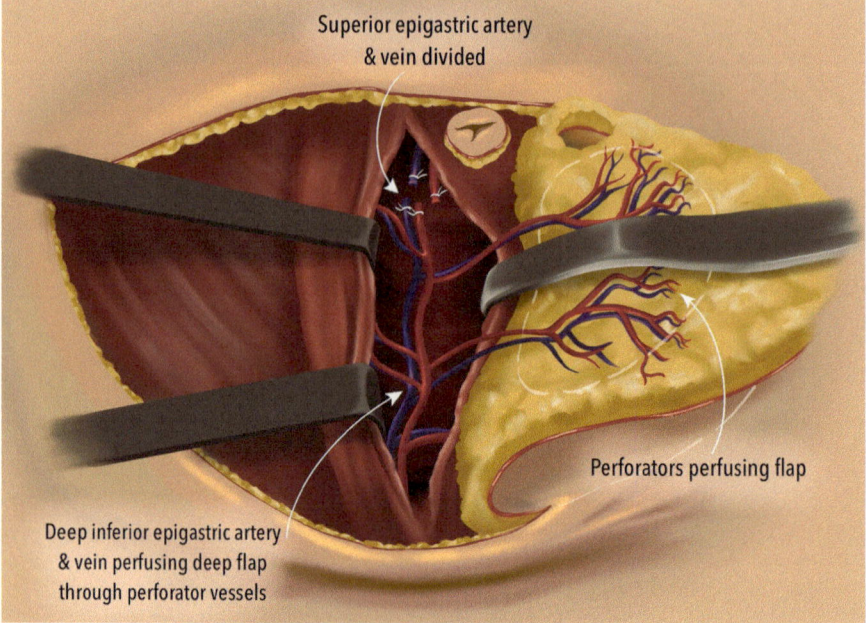

Figure 4.4 Harvest of a deep inferior epigastric perforator (DIEP) free flap.

The skin and fat below the umbilicus and above the pubic area (i.e., the same tissue that would be discarded for an abdominoplasty) are harvested for a DIEP Free Flap.

Even during a typical DIEP harvest, a backup plan is necessary in case there is an unexpected problem with perfusion or anatomy. A long incision from the top of the hip above the pubic area to the other hip was made. Healthy yellow fat sprang through the incision. The first backup is using the superficial inferior epigastric artery (SIEA) and vein (SIEV) as the blood supply to the fat and skin of the abdominal wall. These vessels are in the fat and do not course underneath the abdominal wall musculature. Lydia's SIEV was big, 2.5 mm in diameter. It could be used as a backup for additional venous outflow. However, the SIEA was less than 1 mm in diameter, not large enough to provide enough blood supply to the entire half of the abdomen. It was clipped.

A 360-degree incision was made around the belly button to free it from the skin. Fortunately, the belly button has a secondary blood supply coming from the abdomen and coursing through its stalk. It remained pink, floating on its stalk. A second long incision was now made from hip to hip above the detached belly button and connecting laterally on both sides with the inferior incision. The connected incisions outlined the lower abdomen into a large ellipse, which was now divided into two potential flaps by a third incision made right down the middle of the ellipse from the belly button to the pubic area. If one side of the abdomen did not have sufficient or reliable perforators, the other side of the abdomen could be used.

Elevation of the flap begins by the hip. With the glistening fascia overlying the muscles of the abdominal wall indicating your depth, the fat and skin are lifted off the abdominal wall until a perforator (a small red vessel and a blue vessel) are seen piercing the fascia and entering the fat. Your assistant gently suspends the piece of abdominal skin and fat vertically in the air so you can more easily spread your dissecting scissors around these perforators. Then with all of the perforators dissected, you must decide which one or two perforators are the largest. Large is about 1 mm and is often determined by feel. A robust perforator will have its own pulse, which one can feel when compressed between your thumb and index finger. Lydia had two large perforators piercing the lateral edge of the rectus abdominis muscle. Another three perforators, closer to the medial border of the muscle, were temporarily occluded with microvascular clamps to stop their flow. With the flap now perfused just by the two lateral perforators, the color and bleeding of the flap was examined. The skin was pink; the fat was bleeding; the pulse in the perforators could be felt. These would work. The three medial perforators were then permanently divided with clips.

The DIEP flap was originally described for breast reconstruction and named in the early 1990s.[1] The main advantage of a DIEP flap versus a TRAM free flap is that with a DIEP flap, little to none of the rectus fascia or the rectus muscle is harvested. This preserves the strength and integrity of the abdominal wall. There is less chance that a hernia or weakness will occur postoperatively, particularly if the intercostal nerves innervating the rectus muscle are preserved. With a free TRAM flap, typically a large piece of the muscle and a larger strip of fascia are harvested. More perforators can be captured with a free TRAM flap because one does not selectively choose just one or two perforators. This does create a relative advantage comparing a free TRAM flap to a DIEP flap. The greater perfusion of a free TRAM flap reduces the risk of fat necrosis. Without a robust blood supply, fat can partially die, leaving areas of hardness and calcifications within the flap.

An additional advantage of a DIEP flap is that because the pedicle is being dissected out of the rectus muscle, the pedicle becomes longer compared to the pedicle of a free TRAM flap. In breast reconstruction, pedicle length is usually not much of an issue. The IMA and IMV vessels are just under the medial ribs deep to where the breast used to be. The pedicles of both a free TRAM flap and a DIEP flap can easily reach the IMA/IMV vessels for technically easy anastomoses. Vein grafts and additional flap design modifications are not necessary.

Prior to its use in breast reconstruction, head and neck microsurgeons had been doing dissections similar to those for the harvest of DIEP flaps for years. These were not officially called "DIEP flaps". Instead, the emphasis was placed on how to harvest an abdominally based free flap with the longest pedicle possible so that the pedicle could reach the neck without vein grafts. This was typically most important when a free flap was being harvested to reconstruct a scalp defect or skin defect of the cheek. These abdominally based free flaps were often designed with a vertical ellipse along the entire length of the abdomen, instead of a horizontal ellipse below the belly button. To obtain pedicle length, only a small cuff of fascia around the perforator was removed. The perforator was tracked though the muscle, which was separated away from the vessels. The bulk of the muscle was not harvested. The pedicle was now significantly longer, making it easier to tunnel the vessels to the distant recipient blood supply in the neck.

Rarely is a DIEP flap or any other variation of an abdominally based free flap used for head and neck reconstruction in present-day surgery. Typically, an ALT free flap, instead of a DIEP flap, is the preferred flap. The pedicle is longer, and the donor site morbidity is minimal. Though originally described in 1984,[7] the ALT did not become popular until the early 2000s. In fact during my two residencies and fellowship at three major academic institutions from 1992 to 2002, I did not see or participate in the harvest of a single ALT free flap. Other flaps, usually a radial forearm flap, scapular flap, or abdominal flap, were preferred. In 2005 as an attending plastic surgeon at the University of Pittsburgh, I did my first ALT free flap. It was an ALT flap that was harvested and sewn into a tube to replace the throat of a patient who had undergone a total pharyngectomy for oropharyngeal cancer. Thanks to the internet, one could actually search "ALT Free Flap" to see a video of a surgeon performing the surgery. To my knowledge, it was the first ALT free flap done at the University of Pittsburgh Medical Center. A few years later, in 2008, we published our findings regarding the first ALT free flap to be done in a child for a cheek defect after resection of an epitheliod sarcoma.[8]

Lydia's surgery went as planned. The DIEP flap was harvested from the left hemi-abdomen. The fascia and muscle of the abdominal wall were preserved. The DIEA and DIEV were sewn into the IMA and IMV, respectively (Figure 4.5). The perfused DIEP flap was then placed and trimmed to fit in the breast pocket previously occupied by the tissue expander. The reconstructed breast was now soft and mobile. Four days later, Lydia was released from the hospital. She went back to work helping Kurt in the chiropractic practice soon after her surgery. These days, she's hiking and walking, enjoying her grandchildren, and enjoying life.

Recovery after a DIEP flap is more difficult than recovery after a breast implant. The abdomen must now heal, not just the breasts. Postoperative pain and activity are similar to what one would expect after a tummy tuck, especially if the surgeon has harvested little to no facia and rectus muscle. A patient usually walks slightly bent at the waist for the first 1–2 weeks to avoid strain on the abdomen. Drains are present for usually about 7–14 days. ERAS (Enhanced Recovery After Surgery) protocols which promote multimodality pain control, including the liberal use of nonsteroidal anti-inflammatories and decreased narcotics, have hastened recovery. By 6 weeks, most patients are back to their preoperative activity level.

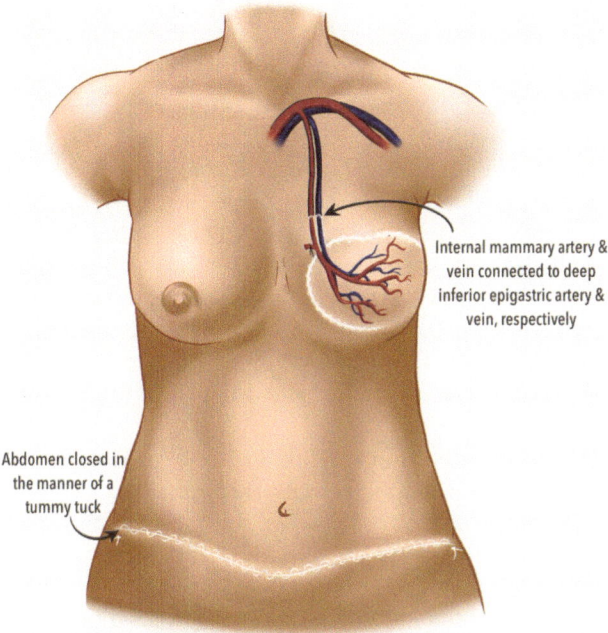

Internal mammary artery &
vein connected to deep
inferior epigastric artery &
vein, respectively

Abdomen closed in
the manner of a
tummy tuck

Figure 4.5 DIEP free flap inset.

The DIEP Free Flap is shaped into a breast mound and its blood vessels are sewn into the IMA and IMV.

There are few scenarios where immediate breast reconstruction is not recommended or discussed. Extreme patient age and the presence of other illnesses, such as severe cardiac or pulmonary disease, may discourage any discussion about reconstruction. More typically, a patient does not receive reconstruction because they do not desire it. They wish to focus on the cancer, treat it, and move on. Having a reconstructed breast is simply not a priority. If it is known before surgery that a patient will likely need radiation after the mastectomy, then single-stage breast reconstruction, such as directly with an implant, is typically not done. Lydia's reconstructive course is more typical. A tissue expander is first placed, and the second stage with autologous tissue is completed after radiation.

However, access to reconstruction, to a plastic surgeon, can also be a hurdle.

Each year, Mrs. B dutifully and apprehensively received an annual 3D mammogram. Both her sister and her aunt had been diagnosed with breast cancer in their 30s. Though a genetic risk, such as a mutation in the BRCA1 or BRCA2 gene, had not been identified, she knew that she probably had an increased risk of breast cancer. Her mammograms always came back as negative, but with the cautionary comment, "breast parenchyma is heterogeneously dense which may obscure small masses." Three months after her last negative mammogram, breast cancer became a reality. A lump in both the right breast and the right armpit could be felt. An MRI confirmed the presence of the breast tumor, and at least four lymph nodes in the axillae appeared likely to contain metastatic cancer. Subsequent biopsies of the breast tumor and the lymph nodes confirmed an invasive ductal breast cancer.

"I told the patient that unfortunately I do not currently have a plastic surgeon who works on Medicaid patients", commented the treating breast surgeon. Mrs. B did not wish to travel 60 miles to the nearest accepting plastic surgeon, so in the winter of 2017, she underwent a modified radical mastectomy without reconstruction. The entire right breast, including the skin, areola, nipple, and axillary lymph nodes were removed. The pectoralis muscle was spared. A 6-week course of radiation therapy to the chest and axilla followed.

In June 2018, I met Mrs. B in consultation for breast reconstruction. The right chest was completely flat, no breast mound, with radiated darkened skin and a scar in the shape of an upside down "T", indicating how the skin had been truncated and closed (Figure 4.6a). The left breast was large, a "DDD", drooping from childbirth and breast feeding in the past. It would have to be reduced and lifted to match any planned reconstruction on the right.

Creating a breast on flat chest is a challenge of volume and surface area. First, the breast boundaries, referred to as the breast footprint, must be marked on the skin. In a unilateral reconstruction the other breast can be used to determine how wide and how tall the breast should be. An abdominal flap, such as a DIEP, is a flat piece of skin and fat. It must be shaped into a conical

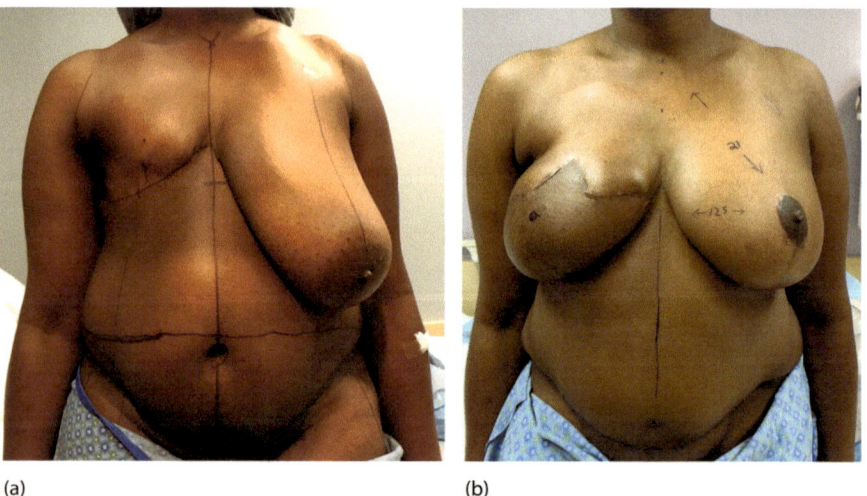

(a)   (b)

Figure 4.6 Mrs. B without reconstruction (a) and after reconstruction (b) with conjoined DIEP free flaps.

mound so that it resembles the natural shape of a breast. Placing a tissue expander at the time of the mastectomy provides important advantages. It preserves the breast footprint and allows the mastectomy skin to be expanded into the shape of a breast. It makes the subsequent autologous reconstruction much easier. The DIEP flap can be used to simply fill the space occupied by the expander. Less skin and intra-op contouring of the flap are needed.

Mrs. B did not have the advantages offered by a tissue expander. If a breast has been cut off, removing all excess skin, a DIEP flap often will not provide enough skin to match a contralateral breast, especially if it is a large breast (Figure 4.6a). A breast reduction on the contralateral breast may solve this problem. However, two flaps are often used, typically 2 DIEP flaps using the majority of the lower abdominal skin and fat. These flaps are either stacked on top of each other to provide additional volume or left connected (i.e., conjoined) without dividing the midline to provide additional skin. The pedicle of each free flap is anastomosed to provide independent blood supply to each flap, and if left without dividing the midline, to provide also augmented (i.e., "supercharged") blood supply to both flaps.

The T-shaped scar on Mrs. B's chest was incised. Radiated skin always seems to bleed more. The underlying pectoralis muscle was stiff, more yellow than pink. Radiation has done its job. With the mastectomy skin elevated off the muscle and lifted to the level of the superior height of the breast, the cavity sprung open. It was massive, the size of a football. Both DIEPs would be needed to replace the missing skin and match the other breast, even after the planned breast reduction.

Providing blood supply to the planned two pedicles now is the main technical challenge. The medial portion of the third rib was removed, and the intercostal muscles between the second and fourth ribs was resected to visualize the underlying IMA and IMV. Divided and with sufficient length, they could now be flipped up and sewn in both an antegrade and retrograde fashion. Arteries will always have an antegrade flow away from the heart, but they can also have backfill (i.e., retrograde flow) from collateral arteries that feed back into the main artery. This backfill is always weaker than antegrade flow, but retrograde flow from an IMA is quite strong and can reliably perfuse a flap. Multiple collaterals between veins also allow reliable venous drainage when connecting into a retrograde IMV.

Without dividing the midline, the conjoined flaps (Figure 4.7) were now transferred to the chest. Inferiorly, a wedge of skin was removed, and sutures were passed through the superficial fascia of the conjoined flaps like purse strings. The sutures were tightened, drawing the tissue together into a conical shape. Both DIEA/DIEV pedicles were draped across the medial chest, and the four vessels were anastomosed antegrade and retrograde into the IMA and IMV. With the flap wells perfused, the conjoined flap was sewn down to the chest wall following the outline of the breast footprint. Along the inframammary fold of the breast, sutures were thrown to intentionally bunch extra skin to accentuate a conical shape and natural breast ptosis.

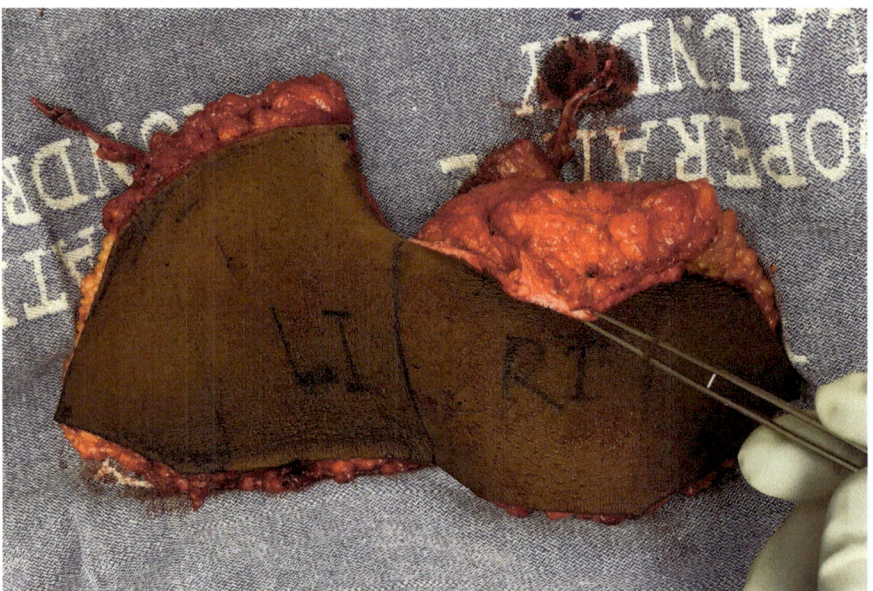

Figure 4.7 Harvest of conjoined DIEP free flaps.

The conjoined flap has 2 separate pedicles which are sewn into each end of the divided internal mammary artery and vein. This allows reliable perfusion of an extremely large flap to replace an entirely missing breast.

Three months later, Mrs. B underwent a left breast reduction to match the right breast reconstruction.

When she was last seen 3 years after her conjoined flaps, Mrs. B was cancer free. She was delighted with her breast reconstruction. The breasts matched in volume and shape (Figure 4.6b). She no longer had the upper neck pain that she associated with her large breasts prior to surgery.

When I asked Mrs. B if there was any advice that she would like to offer to other patients, she responded:

> Do not allow your mind to give into your sickness. I have let God guide me. Every day that he has given me, I have done my best. You need to ask yourself what is the goal that you want to achieve.

Mrs. B's journey through her breast reconstruction clearly raises issues of access and variability of care. Breast reconstruction rates vary widely by location. A 2014 study published in the *Journal of Clinical Oncology* found that in North Dakota, 18% of women choose to have reconstruction, versus 80% living in Washington, D.C.[9] The authors of the study attributed this variation to the number of plastic surgeons living and working in the area.

However, what is harder to capture and explicitly describe is the surgeons' perspective on their clinical practice.

Multiple surveys have indicated that plastic surgeons prefer implant-based reconstruction. The fact that approximately 80% of breast reconstruction is done with implants versus 20% with autologous reconstruction underscores this preference. This bias remains even though the improved quality of life of autologous reconstruction is well known. Lack of microsurgical expertise, time spent in the operating room, and poor insurance reimbursement negatively influence the availability of autologous reconstruction.[10] Moreover, every surgeon has an inherent bias in their practice based on their expertise.

A plastic surgeon needs to have all tools at his/her disposal. If a particular plastic surgeon is not an experienced microsurgeon, a balanced discussion of the relative advantages and/or disadvantages of autologous reconstruction may be lacking. Whether a patient actually makes a high-quality decision about breast reconstruction depends on this balanced discussion.

Surgeons have routinely raised the concern that the physician payment relative to effort may constrain their ability to perform microvascular surgery. Physicians are compensated according to work relative value units (wRVUs). Every medical act and procedure, those actions that physicians take on a daily basis to care for their patients, is distinctively identified by individual current procedural terminology (CPT) codes and is also assigned a number of wRVUs. To convert the relative value calculation into an actual dollar amount, a national conversion factor is implemented. The conversion factor is adjusted annually by the Center for Medicare and Medicaid (CMS) Services to maintain budget neutrality. Payments are not determined by individual case specifications, nor even by clinical outcomes. Rather, physician payment is determined by the procedural codes submitted for reimbursement to the insurance carriers. For the same code, government-funded insurance routinely provides decreased reimbursement compared to commercial carriers. It is the expectation of the federal Medicare system that these wealthy payers in a diverse case mix will buffer the cases in which physician payments are poor. However, not all surgeons accept Medicare or Medicaid insurance. This often skews the poorest-paying and most difficult cases to those surgeons that do accept all patients regardless of insurance.

The CPT code 19364 for breast free flap is the code accepted by CMS and the majority of commercial carriers. However, some commercial payers may accept Health Care Procedure Coding System (HCPCS) S codes. These S codes were originally requested by Blue Cross/Blue Shield for a variety of procedures, devices, and drugs. Though they are listed by CMS, CMS does not routinely reimburse for S codes. The S code S2068 describes breast reconstruction with deep inferior epigastric perforator flap (DIEP) or superficial inferior epigastric artery flap. There is no public list of the insurance carriers, states, regions, or surgeons who are billing and accepting code S2068 instead of CPT code 19364. Surgeons will argue that CPT code

19364 is a generic breast free flap code that includes other abdominal free flaps requiring less work and expertise.

Even though in many cases the same microvascular procedure is being performed, the surgeon billing with S codes will be reimbursed considerably more. For example, using the Massachusetts All-Payer Claims database, one study in 2021 reported a 2.7-fold increase in payments using S codes for breast free flap.[11] The median reimbursement per wRVUs was $321.61 for S code S2068 versus $121.54 for CPT code 19364. The wRVUs assigned to a breast free flap is 42.6 wRVUs. Thus, median total payment to the surgeon was $13,700 for S code S2068 versus $5,178 for CPT code 19364. This vast difference in payment is likely one of the main reasons why women with governmental insurance have a lower probability of undergoing autologous reconstruction compared to women with commercial insurance.

Besides, from S codes, there is no consistent or significant difference between the median payment per wRVU for the remainder of breast reconstructive procedure. CPT codes for tissue expander (i.e., CPT code 19357: median payment, $129.6 per wRVU) and implant reconstruction pay statistically the same amount compared to the widely used free flap breast code, CPT 19364 (median payment: $121.53 per WRVU). In 2021, the wRVUs assigned to a breast tissue expander (CPT code 19357) was 18.5 wRVUs. Thus, the total payment to the surgeon for a unilateral tissue expander is estimated to be $2,397.

Payment per hour is perhaps a better estimate of perceived value. Consider that placement of breast tissue expander takes only 1–1.5 hours of surgeon time, whereas a DIEP flap takes routinely 4–6 hours. A DIEP free flap reconstruction also includes a hospital admission and typically 3–5 days of daily rounding. There is no additional payment for this postoperative care for the next 90 days. This translates into a considerable, relative financial advantage of performing implant reconstruction. For example, in a comparison of breast reconstruction procedures done at the University of Michigan, physician reimbursement by the hour in the operating room was nearly fourfold higher for placing an immediate tissue expander ($1,622 per hour) compared to delayed DIEP or SIEA free flap ($435 per hour).

Comparing microsurgery of the breast to microsurgery of other parts of the body, breast microsurgical breast reconstruction pays more. This is particularly true in comparison to head and neck reconstruction. In 2007, we published the physician and hospital financial reimbursements for 58 consecutive patients with head and neck cancer who were reconstructed with a free flap.[12] The mean actual payment to the surgeon for a free flap was $2,300. Reimbursement for a free flap if a patient was enrolled in medical assistance (e.g., Medicaid) was $993. Remember, these complex head and neck microsurgical reconstructions routinely involve 6–10 hours of work. There is no clear explanation for the relatively greater payments for breast microsurgery procedures. A larger number of head and neck cancer patients are older, with Medicare as the primary payer. Relatively fewer patients have affluent, commercial insurance.

Given the prevalence of breast cancer and the demand for autologous reconstruction, especially among more affluent and educated patients, some plastic surgeons may be in a position to negotiate better contracts for themselves or for their health care systems by offering microvascular reconstruction.

There are other attractive features of breast reconstruction compared to other microsurgical cases. Head and neck microsurgical operations are often considered more technically challenging than some breast microsurgical operations. In head and neck reconstruction, there is a greater range of flaps that the surgeon must master. Breast microsurgical cases have greater case predictability. Mastectomy defects, especially if a tissue expander was placed first, are relatively well defined, whereas a head and neck defect can involve multiple sites of the face, mouth, and/or throat. With a DIEP flap, the harvest routinely begins first thing in the morning, whereas with some head and defects one needs to wait until the tumor has been removed later in the day. Patients with head and neck cancer have worse overall medical health with high rates of cardiovascular and pulmonary disease and malnutrition. Postoperative care in the hospital is longer, usually 7–14 days, and more complex with the need for multiple services to help with medical management. Complications in head and neck reconstruction are much harder to manage. If a DIEP flap fails, the flap can be removed, often with closure of the breast defect. One can then allow the patient to be discharged with a subsequent reconstructive plan in the following weeks to months. If a head and neck free flap fails, the patient will likely need immediate additional flap surgery while in the hospital to prevent catastrophic infections and long-term dysfunction in eating, speaking, and appearance.

Surgical centers, both in private and academic practices, now exist that offer only breast reconstruction. Implant reconstruction will likely be offered by multiple plastic surgeons within most communities. Thus, the marketing for these centers typically focuses on emphasizing autologous reconstruction with the availability of experienced microsurgeons. Given the decreased reimbursement, many of these centers will not accept government insurance and will limit their acceptance of commercial insurance if it also pays poorly. Obviously, patient flow through a health system and access to autologous reconstruction should not be influenced by insurance status. However, it is.

The gap between medicine being a noble possession and the reality that it is a business can be discouraging. Given the low reimbursement for a free flap, especially for a non-breast free flap, and the competing option of pursuing higher-paying surgery, few plastic surgeons may choose to devote themselves to microvascular surgery. Thus, how can physicians pursue higher reimbursements so that they can become financially motivated (and financially solvent) to devote themselves to microsurgery?

Contract negotiations between the physician and insurance company are one option. However, physicians traditionally have had less bargaining power with insurance companies than with hospitals. The service of microvascular reconstruction provides a robust revenue stream for the hospital. In our study of the previously mentioned head and neck cancer patients, payments to the hospital for 58 patients totaled $2,765,552.[12] After covering direct costs, hospital revenue (i.e., margin) was $1,056,886. On the other hand, the mean actual payment to the surgeon for a free flap was $2,300. Institutional awareness of the financial advantage of microvascular surgery should provide an internal incentive to the hospital for a change to physician reimbursement. Without the service of free-tissue transfer, the hospital would lose substantial revenue. For their mutual benefit, hospitals could join with physicians in contract negotiations with the insurance companies. Renegotiated contracts would give surgeons additional incentive to take on such intense cases. Without the service of free-tissue transfer, patients with cancer would receive less-than-optimal reconstructive care.

Surgeons should examine their own practices, especially if they are in the context of a large tertiary hospital, and should determine how their clinical activities contribute to the financial well-being of the institution. Such activities should maintain the financial solvency not only of the hospital but also of the physician. Bolstered reimbursement figures would better attract and retain skilled microsurgeons and still create tremendous revenue for the institution. Given a dedicated surgeon base that agrees to perform large numbers of free-flap procedures, a "center of excellence" within a tertiary care institution could be developed.

Numerous articles have addressed the importance of centers of excellence and volume in ensuring quality outcomes, such as a shorter length of stay, lower rates of morbidity and mortality, and decreased costs. High-volume hospitals have been shown to have better outcomes in large part because patients at these hospitals are likely to be treated by high-volume surgeons. The mechanism for these improved outcomes may be the judgment and technical skill that is gained from frequently performing a particular procedure. Improved outcomes may also reflect appropriate structural characteristics and formalized processes of care within the system. Important structural components at the system level would include critical-care staffing familiar with the postoperative care of free-flap patients, the availability of diagnostic technology, and other resources such as rehabilitation facilities and personnel (i.e., nurses, intensivists, oncologists) experienced with the care of cancer patients.

Successful outcomes for cancer patients can be potentially ensured if surgeons remain devoted to reconstructive microsurgery. Ultimately, individual microsurgeons will choose their practice area based on intellectual and personal values, not necessarily influenced just by economic concerns. Surgeon and author Allen Richard Seltzer astutely wrote, "You are in the service to your patient, and a servant should know his place".[13] Plastic surgeons who have devoted their practice to microsurgery serve patients with life-altering diagnoses that need complex care that few surgeons can provide. Our place is to provide this care, but we must also advocate for our patients while understanding the economics involved.

REFERENCES

1. Allen RJ, Treece P. Deep inferior epigastric perforator flap for breast reconstruction. *Ann Plast Surg* 1994;32:32.
2. Granzow JW, Levine JL, Chiu ES, Allen RJ. Breast reconstruction with the deep inferior epigastric perforator flap: history and an update on current technique. *Journal of Plastic, Reconstructive & Aesthetic Surgery* 2006;59:571–579.
3. American Society of Plastic Surgeons. *2022 Plastic Surgery Statistics Report*, September 26, 2023 (https://www.plasticsurgery.org/plastic-surgery-statistics-2022).
4. Pusic AL, Matros E, Fine N, Buchel E, Gordillo GM, Hamill JB, Kim HM, Qi J, Albornoz A, Klassen AF, Wilkins EG. Patient-reported outcomes 1 year after immediate breast reconstruction: results of the Mastectomy Reconstruction Outcomes Consortium Study. *J Clin Oncol* 2017 Aug 1;35(22):2499–2506.
5. Santosa KB, Chen X, Qi J, Ballard TNS, Kim HM, Hamill JB, Bensenhaver JM, Pusic AL, Wilkins EG. Postmastectomy radiation therapy and two-stage implant-based breast reconstruction: is there a better time to irradiate? *Plast Reconstr Surg.* 2016 Oct;138(4):761–769.
6. Emery E. After a mastectomy, she had breast reconstruction without implants. *UCHealth Today*, May 3, 2019 (https://www.uchealth.org/today/breast-reconstruction-without-implants).
7. Song YG, Chen GZ, Song YL. The free thigh flap: a new free flap concept based on the septocutaneous artery. *Br J Plast Surg* 1984 Apr;37(2):149–159.
8. Nayak JV, Teot LA, Vyas Y, Snyderman CH, Toh EH, Deleyiannis FW. Head and neck epithelioid sarcoma in a child: diagnostic dilemma and anterolateral thigh free flap reconstruction. *Int J Pediatr Otorhinolaryngol.* 2008 May;72(5):719–724.
9. Reshma J, Jiang J, Momoh AO, Alderman A, Giordano SH, Buchholz TA, Kronowitz SJ, Smith BD. Trends and variation in use of breast reconstruction in patients with breast cancer undergoing mastectomy in the United States. *J Clin Oncol* 2014;32(9):919–926.
10. Sando IC, Chung KC, Kidwell KM, Kozlow JH, Malay S, Momoh AO. Comprehensive breast reconstruction in an academic surgical practice: an evaluation of the financial impact. *Plast Reconstr Surg.* 2014 Dec;134(6):1131–1139.
11. Shamsunder MG, Sheckter CC, Sheinin A, Rubin D, Berlin NL, Mehrara B, Matros E. Variation in payment per work relative value unit for breast reconstruction and nonbreast microsurgical reconstruction: an all-payer claims database analysis. *Plast Reconstr Surg.* 2021 Mar 1;147(3):505–513.
12. Deleyiannis FW, Porter AC. Economic factors affecting head and neck reconstructive microsurgery: the surgeons' and hospital's perspective. *Plast Reconstr Surg.* 2007 Jul;120(1):157–165.
13. Selzer R. *Letters to a Young Doctor.* Simon & Schuster, 1982, p. 53.

Chapter 5

Guns

The long-term damage after the shooting stops

Someone should tell self-important anti-gun doctors to stay in their lane.

> – Tweet from the National Rifle Association (NRA),
> November 7, 2018

Do you have any idea how many bullets I have pulled out of corpses weekly? This is not just my lane. It's my f****** highway!

> – Tweet in response: forensic pathologist Judy Melinek

Put her hand into someone's face, into a bloody soup of teeth, bone, and flesh. Self-inflicted gunshot wounds eventually all begin to appear tragically the same. There is an entry point of the bullet below the chin. The mandible has been blown apart into multiple bony pieces with the teeth now free-floating in the mouth. The bullet, often now broken into several metallic shards, pierces the palate, and either exits through the cheek, nose, or eye. Penetration through the nose or eye into the brain often leads to death.

I have been in the unfortunate position to care for patients who are the victims of attempted suicide or homicide, or who have suffered other grievous injuries from firearms. Gun violence is like cancer. As the number of guns in the United States increases, like advanced cancer destroying the healthy, gun violence has become more prevalent and deadly, affecting all aspects of normal life. Children and parents worry about gun violence and mass shootings at school. Verbal disagreements or perceived acts of disrespect end with the brandishing of a gun. Somehow, politicians argue that there should be no limitations, red flag laws, gun safety training, or mental health assessment before an individual purchases a gun. Mythical "good guys with guns" are seriously offered as one solution to combat gun violence. Some have posted cards of their family posing with their collection of guns before their festive Christmas tree and signs of their faith. Recently, one, former Missouri governor Eric Greitens, went so far as to produce a campaign video showing himself leading a group of heavily armed men in tactical gear.[1] They burst into a hypothetical home hunting for persons not true to their political beliefs. I guess that they were the "good guys with guns"?

 DOI: 10.1201/9781003538028-6

Having trained in England and continental Europe, I have never been able to offer a coherent or logical response to my non-US colleagues why the United States allows such a cancer, gun violence, to spread relatively unchecked and untreated. Political ads featuring guns only serve to feed this cancer. To many Americans, proposing limits on guns is akin to proposing limits on who they are and what they should believe. To some, Jesus, Guns, and the Constitution are somehow stitched together in a quilt of righteousness. In June 2022 at a Christian conference in Colorado Springs, one polarizing and conspiring-throwing politician, Rep. Lauren Boebert (R-CO), told a joke that began with the following: "on Twitter, a lot of the little Twitter trolls like to say, 'Oh, Jesus didn't need an AR-15, how many AR-15s do you think Jesus would've had?'". She continued: "Well, he didn't have enough to keep his government from killing him".[2] One even more depressing aspect of American gun culture is how totally dissociated it is from any skill standard. For example, as of September 1, 2021, Texans can carry a handgun without a license or any training.[3] Can you imagine a similar law allowing a surgeon or anyone who wishes to wield a knife to cut into you without a medical license or training?

Ten years after nearly being assassinated by John Hinckley Jr, President Ronald Reagan (1911–2004), a Republican and proud member of the National Rifle Association (NRA), wrote in a March 29, 1991, editorial for *The New York Times* that "this level of violence must be stopped".[4] In the opinion piece, Reagan endorsed the Brady Bill that was being considered in Congress to establish federal background checks of firearm buyers for criminal records or for known histories of mental disturbances. The Brady Bill, which became the Brady Law in 1993 partially because of President Reagan's support, was named after Jim Brady (1940–2014), Reagan's press secretary.[5] In 1981 during the attempted assassination of President Reagan, Jim Brady was permanently disabled. The bullet entered the left side of Brady's forehead and passed through his brain before it exited the right side of the skull. He was left with brain damage, slurred speech, chronic pain, and a partial paralysis that required full-time use of a wheelchair. Reagan commented, "this might never have happened if legislation that is before Congress now – the Brady bill – had been the law back in 1981".

After the Brady Bill was initially proposed, the NRA mobilized and spent millions trying to defeat the legislation. Numerous concessions were obtained, including the replacement of the five-day waiting period of handgun sales for an instant computerized background check and the lack of any regulation (i.e., background check) on the huge secondary market of acquiring guns from unlicensed sellers. The NRA funded numerous lawsuits arguing that the Brady Act was unconstitutional. These eventually led to the US Supreme Court reviewing the case of *Printz v. United States*, 521 U.S. 898. In the 1997 decision in the case, the Supreme Court determined that the provision of the Brady Law that required local law enforcement to conduct background checks was a violation of the Tenth Amendment of the Constitution.

The Tenth Amendment, part of the Bill of Rights, expresses the principle of federalism, or states' rights, by stating that the federal government only has those powers delegated to it by the Constitution. All other powers not forbidden to the states are reserved to each state. According to the Supreme Court decision, local and state law officials remained free to conduct background checks if they so choose, but this could not be mandated by the federal government. The Brady Law remained largely intact except for the federal mandate. Presently, the vast majority of state and local enforcement agencies comply with the background checks as outlined in the Brady Law.

No less important was President Reagan's support in 1994 for a ban on assault rifles. In a joint letter to all House members, Presidents Gerald R. Ford, Jimmy Carter, and Reagan expressed their support for the ban and joined with President Bill Clinton in his campaign against the sale of assault weapons and large-capacity magazines, defined as those that could carry more than 10 rounds.[6] In their joint letter, they said: "This is a matter of vital importance to the public safety. … Although assault weapons account for less than 1% of the guns in circulation, they account for nearly 10% of the guns traced to crime". The ban did pass, but in a final compromise, it was limited to 10 years. It expired in 2004 after Congress let it lapse.

Ronald Reagan, perhaps more than any other politician, understood the devastation of gun violence because he was a victim. Patti Davis, his daughter, recently wrote that

> On the day my father was released from the hospital after John Hinckley nearly killed him, … the world saw him confident, unafraid. What you didn't see was the Secret Service putting a bullet proof vest on him in the hospital room, carefully strapping it over the long incision on his chest.[7]

It is these hidden wounds that surgeons treat and see every day in America. The majority of the public sees only glimpses of this devastation. Gun violence has not stopped, as President Reagan wished. It has only gotten worse.

The best medical training for treating the victims of gunshot wounds (GSWs) is now no longer serving in the military but instead working in a Level 1 trauma hospital in the United States. Many Level 1 trauma hospitals report treating 20 to 40 GSWs per month. Following the COVID-19 outbreak, these rates have only increased. Rising rates of unemployment, socioeconomic stress, domestic abuse, and family violence are the often-quoted reasons. However, an important reason for this violence is the obvious: guns are everywhere, and anyone can get one.

The morning of July 20, 2012, began like any other day. At 5:00 a.m., I turned on the national news and jumped on the treadmill to begin a morning workout. Another mass shooting: police cars and ambulances filled the TV screen. Squad cars had already transported some victims to nearby hospitals. Dozens had been shot and likely killed. A crazy with his hair dyed orange and calling himself the "joker" had been arrested. And then I saw the location: Century 16 Multiplex at the Town Center at the Aurora shopping mall. Aurora, Colorado? Yes, Denver. My medical center was one of the closest hospitals, if not the closest hospital, to the shooting. I jumped off the treadmill and drove immediately to the hospital.

The so-called "joker" fired 76 shots in the theater: 65 from a semi-automatic assault rifle, 6 from a shotgun, and 5 from a .40-caliber Glock handgun. Seventy people were hit with bullets with 12 victims dying, 10 at the scene and 2 more in local hospitals.[8] As a plastic surgeon, I did not expect to be on the front line triaging patients as they were being resuscitated and rushed into the Emergency Department. My role would inevitably be taking care of those patients who survived but were now missing chunks of flesh destroyed by a bullet.

A penetrating bullet transfers a destructive cone of energy to the surrounding tissue. The impact creates a pressure wave that moves perpendicular to the path of the bullet, accelerating tissue forwards and sideways. This creates a temporary cavity up to 30 times the original cross-sectional area of the bullet. This cavity quickly collapses on itself. A smaller permanent pathway marked by blackened dead tissue, hemorrhage, bullet fragments, and sometimes bone chips is left behind. Some percentage of the surrounding tissue affected by the cavitation, the shock waves, will inevitably die. This injury is directly related to the amount of kinetic energy transferred to the tissue. The equation $E = \frac{1}{2}mv^2$, where E is the kinetic energy, m is the mass of the bullet, and v is the velocity of the bullet, quantitates this destructive energy. The tissue-damaging capacity of a bullet is thus most directly related to its velocity. A typical handgun muzzle velocity runs from about 750 FPS (feet per second) to 1,300 FPS and produces a pathway of tissue destruction in the order of 1–2 inches. On the other hand, rifle velocities generally run from 1,900 FPS to 4,000 FPS. The bullet fired from a rifle will literally pulverize the surrounding tissue, much like a watermelon being thrown onto concrete from a height. Assault rifles, such as the AR-15, are designed to shoot more accurately and rapidly than a typical hunting rifle. They have less recoil, which allows rapid firing and can carry large-capacity ammunition magazines which permit 30 or more bullets into the rifle without reloading. They are designed to hunt people, to kill people, not animals.

After the Aurora shooting, Christopher Nolan, director of *The Dark Knight Rises*, the movie that was being played in the theater where the shooting occurred, released a statement on behalf of the cast and crew of the film. It expressed the "profound sorrow of the senseless tragedy" and explained the "the movie theater is my home."[9] No blame was cast on the crew or actors playing the Batman or the Joker. It was the fault of a depressed, deranged, possibly psychotic individual. Nolan's statement continued: "nothing any of us can say could ever adequately express our feelings for the innocent victims of this appalling crime". Indeed, words do become meaningless when you try to describe the devastation caused by guns. They are not personal enough. The public should see and actually feel this

physical and emotional damage. Without this raw confrontation, gun violence remains something to be indirectly debated, something about "sacred"
Second Amendment rights that should not be infringed even if it means
more violence, more guns, and more death.

Allow me, as a plastic surgeon, to express how someone's sense of security, sense of home, and right to live safely are destroyed by guns. Let me
show you how they destroy tissue and how difficult reconstruction can be.
People are never the same, physically or emotionally, after they have been a
victim of gun violence.

The bullet, fired from the "joker's" Smith & Wesson M&P Assault Rifle
15, pierced Jessica's (the name has been changed) right leg, blowing a hole
through the tibia (i.e., the shin bone), the main weight-bearing bone of the
lower extremity (Figure 5.1). The charred hole with blackened edges marked
the likely entry point of the bullet. It was small, less than an inch on the
posterior aspect of the calf. The anterior shin had a 12-cm tear in the skin
with exposure of the underlying fractured tibia. The bullet had shattered
into multiple fragments after pulverizing the bone. The fragments of bullet
and bone were now lodged in the calf muscles. Most of the soft tissue
surrounding the comminuted, tibial fracture was pink and bleeding. Perhaps,
plastic surgery would not be needed.

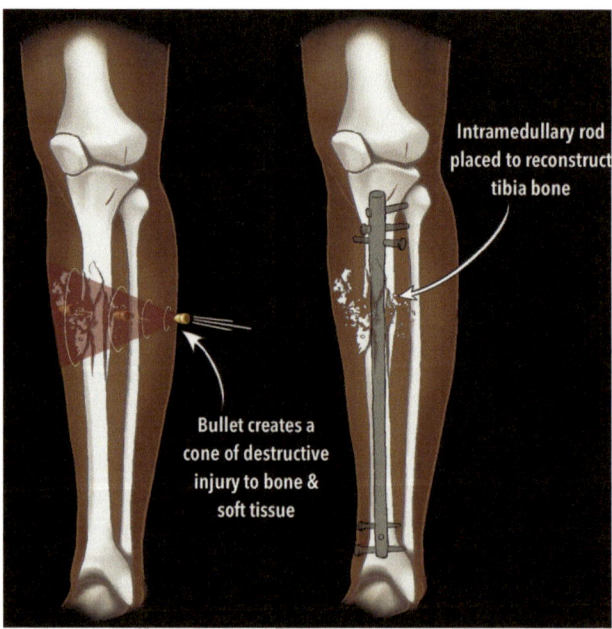

Figure 5.1 Gunshot wound to the lower extremity in a victim of the 2012 Aurora
shooting.

**The bullet entered the right leg, blowing a hole in the tibia and the
surrounding soft tissue.**

To help guide the management of fractures with broken skin (i.e., open or compound fractures), surgeons rely on the Gustilo Anderson classification, also known as the Gustilo classification. Gustilo grades range from I to III, with higher-grade injuries associated with worse soft tissue injury and higher complications. Jessica's open tibial fracture was graded as a Gustilo Type IIIa: an open segmental fracture with extensive soft-tissue injury, but still with adequate soft-tissue coverage of the fracture despite the high-energy trauma. Grade IIIb injuries require free or rotational flap coverage in addition to orthopedic management. Grade IIIc requires vascular repair, flap coverage, and orthopedic management.

Just hours after the shooting, the orthopedic surgery service took Jessica to the operating room. The blackened skin and nonbleeding fat and muscle below were cut away with a scalpel and scissors. Then liters of sterile saline were washed through the wound, rinsing out dirt, bacteria, and bits of free-floating, dead flesh. It is a questionable dogma that a high-velocity bullet, once fired from a gun, is itself sterile. Moreover, the high temperature that the bullet attains after being fired does not sterilize the surrounding tissue where the bullet enters. Rather, gunshot wounds are always contaminated by the matter (i.e., bacteria, pieces of clothing, dead flesh) brought into the wound by the bullet.

With the wound now debrided and cleaned, the orthopedic surgery service then placed an intramedullary (IM) titanium rod into the tibia. From the knee, the IM rod was inserted down the marrow canal of the tibia, crossing the area of the fracture for full-length fixation (Figure 5.1). Screws were then placed on both ends to keep it in position during healing. The entry and presumed exit sites of the bullet were again examined. The skin edges were bleeding and appeared healthy. With the edges pushed and stitched together, the closure did not feel too tight. It appeared that it might heal.

"Dr. D, are you free to come up to the Ortho clinic? Jessica is here. I think we have a wound problem". Four weeks after the shooting, I met Jessica for the first time. A two-inch black scab had replaced the previously closed exit site. We all knew what this meant. This dead skin would be just the tip of the iceberg, with additional dead fat and muscle below the scab. The cavity of destruction created by the bullet's energy had declared itself. The dead tissue was not grossly infected with pus puddling out of the wound, yet infection was just a matter of time. Soft tissue Infection on top of a fractured bone will inevitably lead to a long-term infection of the bone (i.e., osteomyelitis). Long-term antibiotics and additional surgery would be needed. If osteomyelitis is not treated, it will eventually result in an amputation.

The surgery was posted urgently for the next morning. With a knife, I unroofed the eschar. Gray muscle oozed up to the skin edges, and this too was cut away. After 20 minutes of cutting and cleaning, the cavity, now 2 inches deep, led straight down to the bone. Through the gap in the leg, the shaft of the titanium rod within the bone reflected the overhead operating lights.

Jessica's wound was in the upper part of the shin (i.e., upper one-third of the lower leg). This part of the leg has the powerful and beefy muscles of the calf, the gastrocnemius and soleus muscle, nearby. Without dividing their blood supply, as done in a free flap, one can detach these muscles from the Achilles tendon and rotate them across the tibia. This allows a healthy piece of muscle to cover the exposed fracture and hardware. Doing just that, a separate 15-cm incision was made down the inner (i.e., medial) side of Jessica's calf. The cutaneous nerve, the sural nerve, providing sensation to the lateral foot, calf, and ankle was dissected and pushed out of the way. Then the medial half of the gastrocnemius muscle was divided from the Achilles tendon just at the point that the muscle blends into the tendon. A tunnel was created connecting the hole over the tibia with the more medially located muscle. With the muscle passed through the tunnel and sewn over the tibia, a skin graft, the size of a dollar bill, was harvested from the thigh and sewn on top of the muscle. Over the next few weeks, the skin graft and muscle flap healed. The fractured bone and rod were no longer visible.

Before July 20, before the shooting, Jessica was a cheerful 19-year-old woman with a healthy active life, supporting herself physically and economically with no concerns. After the shooting, pain and anxiety about not being able to work dominated her thoughts. She did not smile in the clinic. Additional surgery, including bone grafts to replace the missing bone and hardware removal to extract screws, were needed. Nine months after the shooting, Jessica was still allowed to bear only 50% of her weight on her right leg, and she had developed an"equinus" contracture of the lower leg. Named after horses (i.e., "equinus") who essentially walk on their toes, an "equinus" deformity describes the position of the foot being held downward. Jessica's "equinus" deformity was likely caused by a combination of injury to the calf muscles from the bullet, the scar introduced by the reconstructive surgery, and the inability to fully walk on the leg and flex the calf during healing. With physical therapy over the next 2 years, this deformity improved. Eventually, she was allowed to completely bear weight on her right leg. However, years after the shooting, with the bones and soft tissue fully healed, Jessica was still left with mild weakness and intermittent pain in her right leg, especially with fast walking and running. Her smile did return, but it seemed forced and practiced.

The lasting effects of a GSW reach far beyond mortality and physical functional impairment. Survivors experience long-term adverse mental and psychological outcomes. Rates of unemployment, substance abuse, depression, anxiety, and post-traumatic stress disorder (PTSD) are all increased compared to the general population. Many victims, like Jessica, with isolated GSWs to the extremities eventually return to their pre-trauma life seemingly well adjusted. Feelings of sadness, despair, and personal insecurity are somehow dampened, buried, and/or controlled. Nearly 12 years after the shooting, Jessica says that talking about the trauma does help. She receives cognitive therapy once a month. The therapy helps her cope with her PTSD; it redirects her mind, but she still has chronic anxiety.

GSWs to the face present a completely different challenge. They cannot be completely hidden even with the best reconstruction. Appearance, speech, chewing, and swallowing are often handicapped forever. Even if they wished to smile, many reconstructed patients lack the muscles and nerves to perform this basic social and identity-confirming function.

A shotgun is often the weapon of choice of men attempting suicide, and these wounds are more often life-altering than life-ending. At the last moment when the trigger is being pulled, the poor man will often flinch, pulling his head back. The dispersed pellets blow the face off, leaving the brain relatively injured, and the young man completely conscious.

Alex (the name has been changed) was such a young man. The paramedics found him at his home after he discharged a 12-gauge shotgun under his chin (Figure 5.2). In their notes, the paramedics recorded: "the teeth are imbedded into the hard palate. The location of the right eye is undetermined; the nose is not visible. He is awake, able to answer only by shaking his head". The mandible, right cheek, right lower lip, right upper lip, chin, and some of the anterior tongue were also missing, blown across Alex's face and into the ceiling. Having been emergently transported to our Level I trauma center, the anesthesiologist on call easily passed an endotracheal breathing (ET) tube through the gaping hole of the face into the trachea. An hour later in the operating room, the ET tube was exchanged for a tracheotomy tube, and I began to pick out teeth, bone, and mangled flesh out his right eye, cheek, and mouth.

To a nonmedical person, surgical management of a gunshot wound to the face likely seems insurmountable. Everything, meaning bone, teeth, muscle, and skin, has been blasted apart into small pieces. The remaining tissue is sick, dying from the blast, not bleeding well because the blood supply is

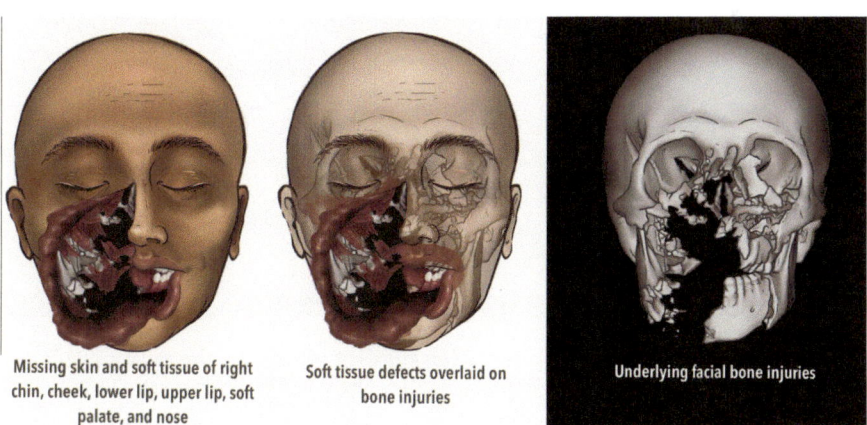

Missing skin and soft tissue of right chin, cheek, lower lip, upper lip, soft palate, and nose

Soft tissue defects overlaid on bone injuries

Underlying facial bone injuries

Figure 5.2 Gunshot wound to the face.

The shotgun blast has removed and destroyed the mandible, midface, and nose. Left – destruction of the soft tissues of the chin, cheek, lips, and nose. Right – destruction of the underlying facial bones.

clotted or destroyed. However, the surgical management becomes much clearer when you simply treat a GSW like a cancer. Cut it all away. Any tissue that is shattered, that is questionably going to heal, cut it away. Then with this tissue gone, rebuild the face just like you would do having removed a cancer.

The next day, we continued to cut and began to rebuild (Figure 5.3). Additional tissue of the cheek, lips, and nose was now no longer bleeding. It was cut away. There was a dime-size hole leading from the nose and sinuses

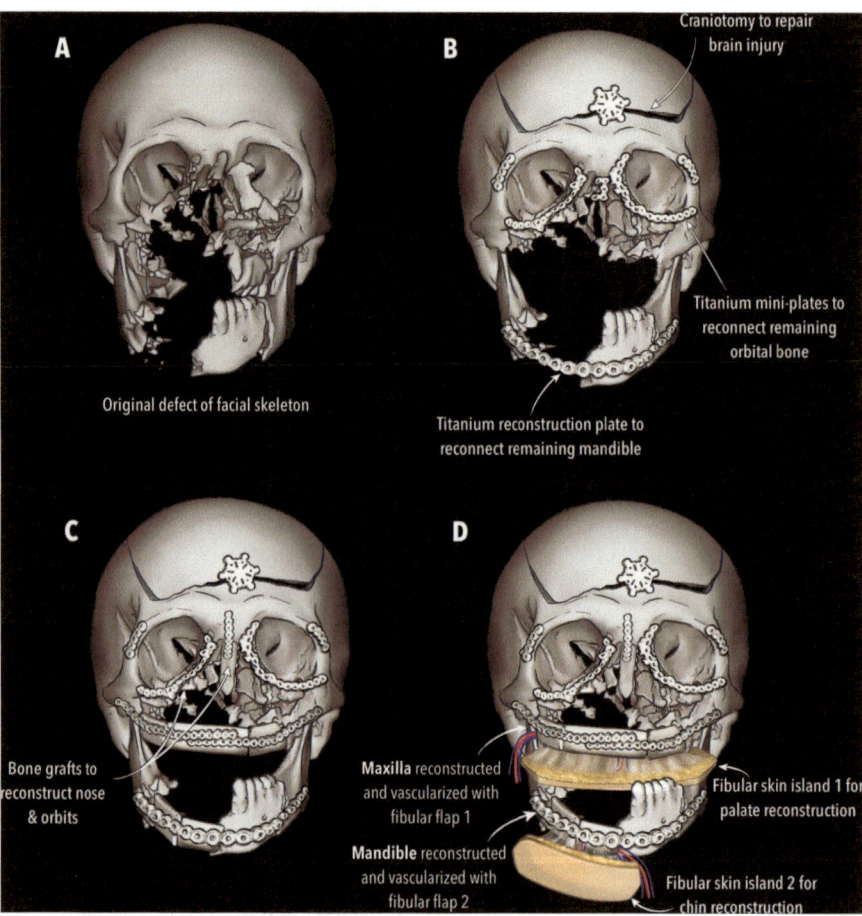

Figure 5.3 Stages of reconstruction after gunshot wound to the face.

Upper right panel (B) – the facial fractures have been reduced and fixated with plates and screws. Lower panels (C and D) – The missing bone of the maxilla and the mandible has been respectively replaced with the first and second fibular free flaps. The skin paddles of the fibular free flaps have been used to replace the soft tissues of the chin, right lower lip, and palate.

into the frontal lobe of the brain. Neurosurgery did a craniotomy to remove the frontal bone, not because the bone was injured, but so the brain could be lifted to expose the hole underneath. With the hole exposed, the dura was repaired to separate the brain from the cavity below containing spit, mucus, and millions of bacteria. With the frontal cranial bone temporarily removed, there now was an opportunity to cut multiple bone grafts from this bone flap. With a saw, I split the inner table of the skull from the outer table. Six domino-size bone grafts were cut from the inner table. One was placed underneath the brain, providing an extra barrier separating the brain from the nose. With the brain debrided, the dura repaired, and the intracranial injury now separated from the face, the frontal bone was then placed back, with plates and screws holding it into position.

Following the same principles that Gilles outlined a century earlier, the reconstruction was then designed from "within outwards". The lining membrane that remained, the mucosa of the mouth and nose, was sewn back into their original positions. The remaining supporting structures of the face – the bones of the cheeks, upper jaw, and nose – were plated into their proper positions with small miniplates of titanium. The bone grafts that had been cut from the skull were used to reconstruct the missing walls of the orbits and to provide support for the nose, since most of these internal nasal structures had been blown away. Now the damage to the mandible was again examined. The central mandible was in dozens of small pieces, with no viable skin or mucosa covering where the chin should have been. Just like a fungating cancer, all of this destroyed tissue was also cut away. Using a saw, I divided the mandible on either side of the blast, removing the mangled bone and soft tissue. A larger titanium reconstruction plate was then plated to the remaining mandibular bone. This restored the continuity of the mandible and some resemblance of a chin. Twelve hours after we started this first major reconstructive step, we stopped (Figure 5.3). The brain was now no longer in gross communication and contamination with the hole in the mouth and the nose. The remaining viable tissue and bone had been placed back into the preexisting positions. However, what remained was now three massive defects: a missing chin; palate; and the right upper lip, cheek, and right lower lip.

To fully treat GSWs to the face, one must be a microsurgeon. Massive wounds with missing skin, muscle, and bone require bringing new, undamaged tissue into the defect. Gilles achieved remarkable success with tubed flaps and multiple, staged surgeries. However, the surgical plan often spanned months and required patients to assume long-term residence at the hospital. In contrast, microsurgery can reconstruct, relatively quickly, nearly any facial defect with much greater certainty, less morbidity, and almost with no limitations. For Alex, 2 days after this first major operation, we used an osteocutaneous fibular free flap from the left leg to replace the missing bones of the central midface, the maxilla and the zygoma (Figures 5.3 and 5.4). The skin paddle of the flap was rotated into the mouth to replace the palate

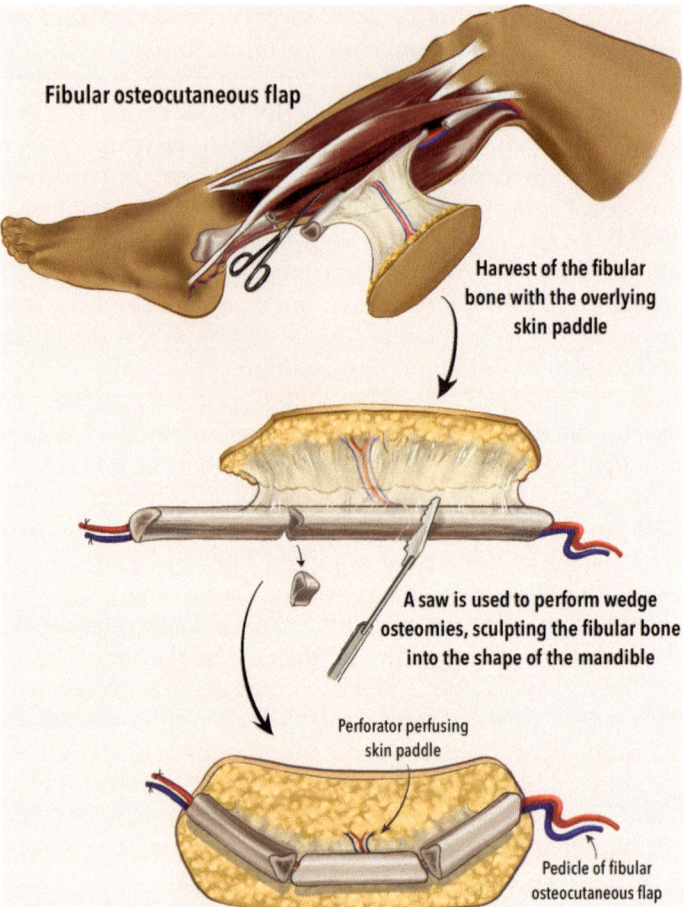

Figure 5.4 Harvest of a fibular osteocutaneous free flap.

The fibular flap based on perfusion from the peroneal artery and veins is harvested with the overlying lateral skin. Osteotomies are done with a saw to bend the straight bone into the shape of the missing bone of the defect.

and upper lip. With the palate reconstructed, Alex's mouth no longer directly communicated with his nose and his eyes. Alex was one step closer to being able to talk and swallow again. Alex's final major surgery occurred just three days later. A second fibular free flap, now from the right leg, was used to replace the mucosa, bone, and skin of the floor of the mouth, mandible, and external chin. An anterolateral thigh free flap was then used to replace the missing tissues of the right lower lip, cheek, and upper lip (Figure 5.5). All three of Alex's free flaps healed well with no complication. Within a few

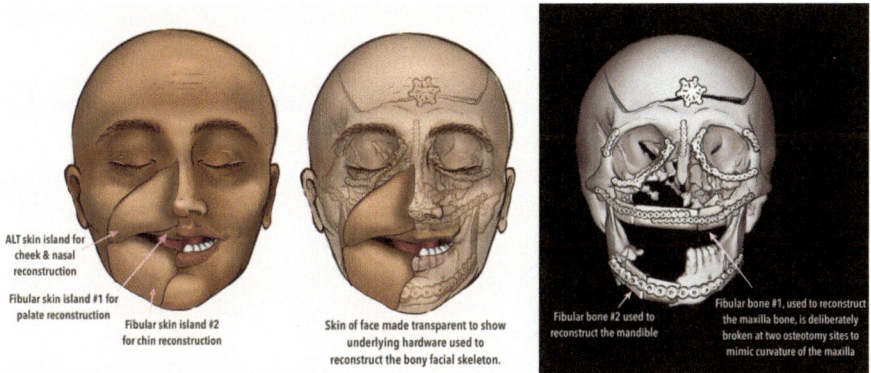

ALT skin island for cheek & nasal reconstruction

Fibular skin island #1 for palate reconstruction

Fibular skin island #2 for chin reconstruction

Skin of face made transparent to show underlying hardware used to reconstruct the bony facial skeleton.

Fibular bone #2 used to reconstruct the mandible

Fibular bone #1, used to reconstruct the maxilla bone, is deliberately broken at two osteotomy sites to mimic curvature of the maxilla

Figure 5.5 Final soft tissue and bony reconstruction of the gunshot wound to the face.

Left – the right cheek has been reconstructed with an ALT Free Flap. The other soft tissue defects of the chin, lips, and palate were reconstructed with the skin paddles of the fibular free flaps. Right – the underlying boney reconstruction with the bone from the fibular free flaps.

weeks, he was taking his entire diet by mouth, and his speech was 100% intelligible.

Though I had spent dozens of hours staring, focusing on Alex's face, I did not initially recognize him a few weeks later at his first clinic visit. It had been 3 months from the date of his GSW and 5 weeks since he had been discharged from the hospital. Dressed in jeans and a long-sleeved work shirt, he looked like any other patient. The anti-COVID masks that all patients and doctors were now required to wear left the eyes as the only revealing facial feature. I saw the sadness and worry in Alex's eyes. I knew it was him. However, with the mask removed, I now saw the gunshot wound, not necessarily Alex.

When facial skin and unique, functionally delicate structures such as the lips and/or the nose are blown off, it is impossible to fully replicate their appearance or function. Free flaps allow tissue to be brought into the wound; they allow the area to heal. They do not allow the face to smile, laugh, speak, breathe, or chew as one did before the gunshot wound. If the facial skin (i.e., the external lining) is relatively intact and just bone and mucosa are missing, free flaps can produce remarkable results. They are hidden underneath normal skin, normal lips, and an existing nose. However, Alex had blown off too many externally facing structures. It was impossible not to see the skin paddles of the three free flaps: one formed the chin, one the cheek and lower lip, and one the palate and the upper lip (Figure 5.5). Only with a mask were these hidden.

Three months later at his next clinical visit, Alex, with his wife and mother present, asked the obvious. "Dr. D, what do you think about a face transplant?" Alex had the type of facial destruction that could be served well by a face transplant.[10] In my opinion, he was a "good surgical candidate". All conventional reconstructive options had been exhausted. He had extensive loss of the central face subunits (i.e., upper and lower lips, nose, and chin) and the associated surrounding skin. His craniofacial reconstruction with bone grafts, plates and screws, and multiple free flaps had allowed him to heal, speak, and eat, but his reconstructed face would always draw stares. Without lips that could purse and completely hold food and liquid in his mouth, he would never get dental implants. From a nonsurgical viewpoint, Alex appeared to have good family and social support. He was under the care of a psychiatrist and did not appear to have any active psychiatric disorder. I discussed with Alex and his family why he might be a good candidate. Patients receiving facial transplantation require mandatory lifelong immunosuppression. We discussed the risks of immunosuppression, ranging from infections to kidney failure and malignancies. They also understood the risk of transplant rejections and the devastating consequence of again having an unreconstructed defect if the face transplant had to be removed.

After this conversation, I listed the few centers in the United States that might offer Alex a face transplant. We discussed that it is still a rare procedure with only about 50 face transplants worldwide having been done. Connie Culp,[11] the first person in the United States to receive a face transplant on December 9, 2008, had been shot in her face by her husband. Face transplants had also been done in multiple patients who had suffered self-inflicted gunshot wounds. Psychiatric care and evaluation were part of the essential screening process. The screening process would undoubtedly focus on whether Alex was still at risk of harming himself. Most people who attempt suicide will not go on to complete suicide. Long-term studies that have followed over time patients who have made suicide attempts that resulted in medical care have shown that approximately 70% never make a second attempt. Suicide crises are often short-lived. However, whether this long-term risk also remains relatively diminished for the subset of victims who have suffered a self-inflicted GSW is unknown. When you cannot hide the effects of self-harm, it is difficult to imagine how one could ever face the world without a continual sense of anxiety, depression, and loss.

Alex and his family did reach out to one of the face transplant centers that we discussed. During his most recent visit, nearly 3 years after his injury, Alex indicated that it was "his ultimate dream" to receive a face transplant. However, my offer to talk to the plastic surgeons that I knew at the center was not greeted with any enthusiasm. Rather, at that moment, Alex wanted to get on with his life, to raise his three children, to be present and available as they grew up. He realized that the screening, surgical preparation, and postoperative care could possibly take him away from his children for an extended period of time. Now was not the time. He was dressed in his work clothes heading back to his landscaping job after today's clinic visit, heading back to his responsibilities as a father. Our conversation will continue as I care for Alex over the coming years.

The long-term damage that gun violence causes will only ever be understood by the people who are the actual victims. It is absolute carnage that can only be exposed at close range. Every advocate of more guns, less training, and less screening should be mandated to somehow visually and viscerally experience the pain of victims. Perhaps they should spend a month following a trauma surgeon, be the person bearing the responsibility to tell a parent that their child has just been shot or be the one holding the knife and cutting away a destroyed body part. Perhaps change will come only as a result of something similar to "Emmett Till moments".[12]

On August 28, 1955, Emmett Till, a 14-year-old African American from Chicago, was brutally murdered for allegedly flirting with a white woman while visiting his family in Money, Mississippi. The assailants, the white woman's husband and brother, beat Emmitt nearly to death, gouged out an eye, and shot him in the head. Three days later, his corpse was found so badly disfigured that it could be identified only by an initialed ring. Mamie Brady, Emmett's mother, requested that the body be sent back to Chicago instead of being quickly buried as the local Mississippi authorities desired. After seeing her son's disfigured body, she wanted the world to see what the racist assailants had done. Over 5 days, more than 100,000 people lined up to see Emmitt's mutilated body, and *Jet* magazine published graphic photographs that were distributed all over the world. Emmett's murder galvanized civil rights workers and widespread outrage against racism. The idea of lawmakers seeing gruesome photos, or more directly actually viewing destroyed bodies, would take away the distance from the reality of gun violence. The arguments for and against such a viewing can be debated from multiple perspectives: from parental consent, to the burden of causing additional mental trauma, to who should have access to a viewing. However, surgeons do not have the luxury of distancing themselves with such a debate. They must step up and actually take care of the victim, not just talk about the problem.

Surgeons are not allowed access to "their lane", to practice their specialty, until they have become board eligible or certified, until they have done enough cases and obtained enough education to do their job safely and well. Activists of gun rights need to earn the right to be in "their lane". In my opinion, this means they should be just as educated as doctors about the physical and mental consequences of gun violence. Every encounter that a surgeon has with a GSW victim is an "Emmett Till moment". Perhaps, lawmakers and gun activists should be "eligible /certified" to voice their opinion about gun laws and restrictions only after they can demonstrate that they have had their own personal moments speaking to victims and touching and seeing a human body ripped apart by a bullet.

After the mass shooting at Robb Elementary School in Uvalde, Texas, on May 24, 2022, in which 19 children and 2 teachers were fatally shot, Shannon Watts (founder of Moms Demand Action) on MSNBC summarized:

> If … you're part of the 50% of America who hasn't been impacted by gun violence, great. Wonderful. It is coming to your community. No one is going to get out of this unscathed. We all have a part to play in changing this dynamic.

We, the surgeons who try to repair the physical damage, have the additional responsibility of exposing gun violence as more than an abstract, distant event. I am confident that nearly every surgeon who treats victims of GSWs would be willing to open "their lane" to any lawmaker or activist interested in seeing this reality. Step up and experience this carnage firsthand. Only then can one really obtain firsthand empathy to contribute to a balanced discussion about guns.

REFERENCES

1. Watson K. Missouri Senate GOP hopeful Eric Greitens hunts political opponents with guns in ad. *CBS News*, June 20, 2022 (https://www.cbsnews.com).
2. Robillard K. Lauren Boebert jokes Jesus could have avoided crucifixion if he'd had AE-15s. *Huffpost*, June 15, 2022 (https://www.huffpost.com).
3. https://guides.sll.texas.gov/Gun-Laws/Carry-of-Firearms.
4. Reagan R. Opinion: Why I'm for the Brady Bill. *The New York Times*, March 29, 1991.
5. Brady Law, Bureau of Alcohol, Tobacco, Firearms, and Explosives (https://www.atf.gov/brady-law).
6. Eaton WJ. Ford, Carter, Reagan push for gun ban. *Los Angeles Times*, May 5, 1994.
7. Davis P. Opinion: my father, Ronald Reagan, taught me a healthy fear of guns. *The New York Times*, July 5, 2022.
8. Willie B, Knowles D. Remembering the victims of the Aurora shooting, 10 years later. *Rocky Mountain PBS*, July 20, 2022.
9. Reuters Staff. "Dark Knight" maker calls shooting "unbearably savage". *U.S. News*, July 20, 2012.
10. Parker A, Chaya BF, Rodriguez-Coloc R, et al. Recipient selection criteria for facial transplantation: a systemic review. *Ann Plast Surg* 2022 Jul 1;89:105–112.
11. Pietsch B. Connie Culp, first face transplant recipient in US, dies at 57. *The New York Times*, August 1, 2020.
12. Evans M. After Uvalde shooting people consider an "Emmett Till moment" to change gun debate. *Los Angeles Times*, June 9, 2022.

Chapter 6

Legacy

What is the main lesson of your life?

> If you would not be forgotten as soon as you are dead, either write something worth reading, or do something worth writing.
> – Benjamin Franklin, 1706–1790

Look back on your own life. You will see all sorts of people who have been legacy leavers to you – parents, teachers, and mentors who have shared lessons and greater truths, such as charity, kindness, and the value of hard work. Legacies come in different shapes and levels of commitment. Financial legacies, such as the support of medical research or donations to institutions, have their place. Yet, the longer-lasting avenues of legacy may be the values and life experiences that we pass and teach to our children, colleagues, mentees, and the greater circle of people with whom we interact.

Ken Dychtwald, PhD, psychologist and gerontologist, has extensively surveyed seniors and their children about what constitutes a meaningful legacy.[1] He writes,

> There's this enormous craving, this desire for people in their maturity to share what they've learned, to pass on lessons of a lifetime, to teach, to feel that their life experience is being invested, even planted, into the field of tomorrow.[2]

Dychtwald continues: "There was also a similar response – a natural, innate appetite on the part of younger generations – to receive that".

In deciding what you want to leave as a legacy, one must consciously look inward. What is the main lesson of your life that you wish to pass on?

A remarkable man, Mr. John C. Lester. "I've never seen a better day!" John's response had been the same nearly every day since his first kidney transplant in 1986. At the age of 21, John had learned that his kidneys were failing due to a rare complication (i.e., post-streptococcal glomerulonephritis) from strep throat. He would continue to lean on that phrase, that optimism, his whole life as he faced the subsequent challenges of health and transplantation. In the summer of 2012, I met John for the first time. His scalp was hairless and bleached from the radiation therapy used to treat the

DOI: 10.1201/9781003538028-7

recurrent skin cancers that had continually resurfaced on his scalp for the last few years. The most recent intervention had removed a large squamous cell carcinoma on his head, leaving a hole the size of a softball. White, dry cortical bone was exposed where the scalp should have been. How could this day be a good day?

Over the next 4 years, our relationship evolved from treating surgeon and patient to friend and mentor. John was a man of formidable strength and optimism. Throughout his life he built an outstanding reputation of success and selflessness. His successful 30-year career was evidence of his character. He served as Director of UBS Wealth Management for Colorado, overseeing a $8.5 billion portfolio and more that 120 financial advisors in seven state-wide offices. No small task for anyone.

In 2001, his first transplanted kidney began to fail. Despite undergoing dialysis treatments three days a week for five hours each day, John continued to work. While he waited for his second kidney transplant, he maintained his top-rated performance with the Western Region for UBS. "And I became a better manager," he said in a *Coloradobiz* interview in 2009:

> When you go through something like that, you become a lot more grounded from a perspective of importance. You have greater ability to empathize with others and recognize that everyone carries a burden of some sort or another. And it's OK that sometimes those things get in the way of our business.[3]

John had made the decision to think differently, to focus on caring for others. His greatest joy on the job was derived from what he called his "psychic income", managing and being around people. I never asked John if he had a "life sentence", a statement that summarized the goals and purpose of his life. However, I suspect that it would have been similar to the following: "I want to pass on hopefulness and confidence about the future so that others can achieve their own goals".

Long-term exposure to immune-suppressive drugs leads to chronic medical conditions, such as post-transplant malignancies, especially of the skin. Immunosuppression inhibits the repair of DNA damaged by ultraviolet (UV) exposure. Some viruses also play a role in causing cases of squamous cell carcinoma, the most commonly occurring skin cancer in renal transplant patients. These viruses transform the skin cells, the keratinocytes, by activation of cancer-promoting genes. With the body's natural immune system damped by immunosuppressive drugs, these potential oncogenic viruses may be reactivated. It has been estimated that 70% of renal transplant patients develop skin cancer after 20 years. Older age, male sex, fair skin type, UV exposure, and the duration of immunosuppression are associated with increasing the risk of a skin cancer. When skin cancers do develop, they are often more aggressive and deadly compared to skin cancers that develop in a non-immunosuppressed patient. They tend to invade blood vessels and nerves, spread to regional lymph nodes, and present with recurrences locally near the site of surgical treatment.

Unprotected areas of skin, especially of the face, scalp, and arms, are where skin cancers are more likely to occur. Accordingly, research has shown that there is a correlation between more time spent driving and a higher incidence of left-sided skin cancer. The left side of the body is more likely to be exposed to the sun while driving. Indeed, John had a number of previous skin cancers excised from his left forearm and now his left scalp. At 5,280 feet above sea level, Denver is known as the Mile High City, which means that persons living in Colorado are some of the most sun exposed in the United States. For every 1,000 feet above sea level, UV exposure increases somewhere between 4% and 10%. Routinely, John and every other Coloradan can enjoy close to 300 days of sunshine a year – or, stated from a cancer perspective, are exposed to 300 days of significantly increased risk of skin cancer.

For transplant patients, immunosuppressive guidelines are designed to create an equilibrium between reducing the risk of transplant rejection and of drug-related adverse effects. There are multiple classes of immunosuppressive drugs including corticosteroids, antimetabolites (i.e., mycophenolic acid, azathioprine), calcineurin inhibitors (i.e., cyclosporine, tacrolimus), mTOR inhibitors (i.e., rapamycin, sirolimus), and biologics (i.e., IL-2, IL-6 inhibitors). Some regimens, such as those that are tacrolimus based versus others that are cyclosporin based, may have a lower risk of promoting skin cancer. After three kidney transplants spanning 26 years, John's immunosuppressive medications had been decreased, adjusted, and changed multiple times. When he finally presented with an aggressive squamous cell of the scalp that had already been treated with radiation therapy, surgery was the only option.

Before the non-adhesive gauze and antibiotic ointment were applied, John's scalp was lovingly washed with baby soap and water each day. Without ointment, the wound would crack, bleed, and ache. I watched as Connor and Tripp, John's two sons, unwrapped the wound. Knowing John's history, the revealed wound was not unexpected (Figure 6.1). It was down to the bone with inflamed, raised edges, indicating cancer was still present. What was gentle and affectionate was that Connor, Tripp, and Erin, John's wife, knew how best to care for John. Graciously, without the aid of me or the nurses, they re-dressed John's scalp, watching his face carefully for any sign of pain.

The surgery would treat the cancer and the open wound by resecting all of the diseased tissue and then replacing it with healthy tissue. The thickness of the skin and fat of the forearm would match well the full thickness of the scalp that had been and was going to be excised. I rotated John's arm to examine the quality of the skin. There were no red, scaly patches to suggest early skin cancers. As I explained the operative procedure of using a right radial forearm free flap (i.e., RFFF) for the scalp reconstruction,

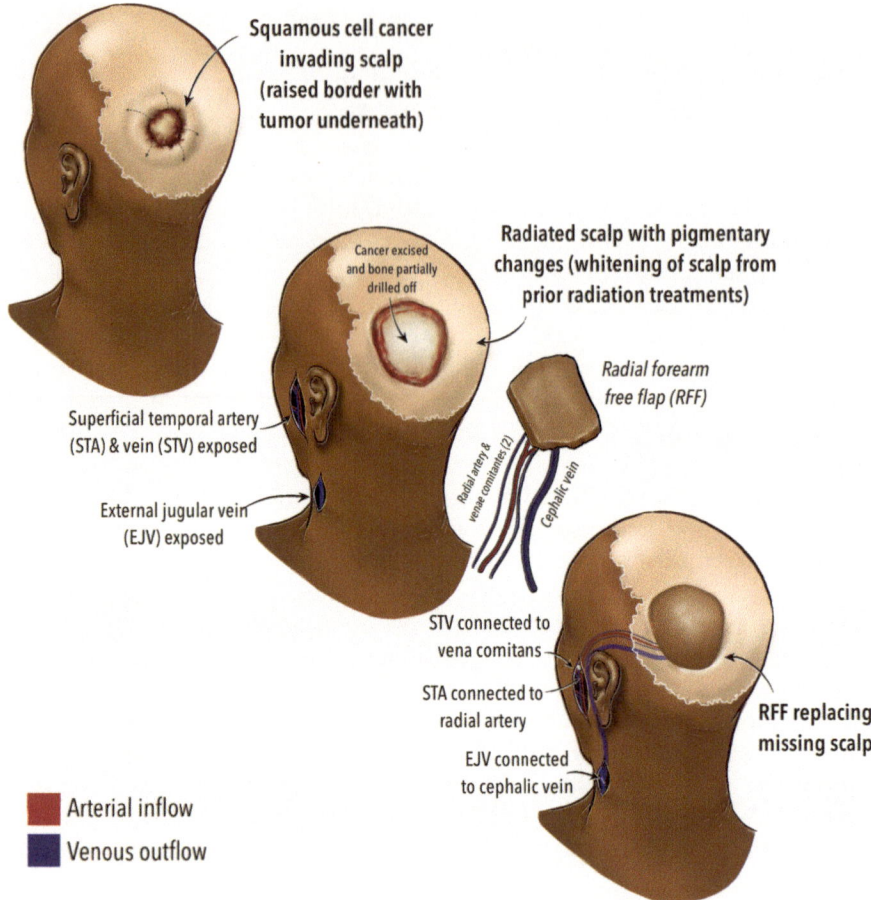

Squamous cell cancer
invading scalp
(raised border with
tumor underneath)

Cancer excised
and bone partially
drilled off

Radiated scalp with pigmentary
changes (whitening of scalp from
prior radiation treatments)

Radial forearm
free flap (RFF)

Superficial temporal artery
(STA) & vein (STV) exposed

External jugular vein
(EJV) exposed

Radial artery &
venae comitantes (2)

Cephalic vein

STV connected to
vena comitans

STA connected to
radial artery

EJV connected
to cephalic vein

RFF replacing
missing scalp

Arterial inflow

Venous outflow

Figure 6.1 The first of four free flaps done over 4 years to treat recurrent skin
cancer, eventually invading into the brain.

**The skin cancer of the scalp is resected leaving the bone of the skull
exposed. The scalp is replaced with a radial forearm free flap that is
sewn into blood vessels in front of the ear.**

John half-jokingly asked, "What about my golf game, will this help my
handicap?" Such a jest told me instantly about John's resilience. I knew that
he would face this difficulty head-on without despair, just like he had done
for his kidney transplants.

It is hard to know where cancer begins and ends after radiation therapy
has been delivered. Thickened, bleached, dry, and irritated, the skin around
John's original skin cancer was not healthy. Asleep in the operating room
and now bathed in Betadine from his scalp to his right arm, John was fully
exposed. Labelled like the hours of a clock, multiple skin biopsies at 1
o'clock, 2 o'clock, etc. were taken in the scalp 2 centimeters away from the

ulcer, the obvious cancer. There were 10 biopsies in total. The pathologist was called into the operating room to show the condition of the radiated scalp and where the biopsies had been taken.

The frozen section refers to a process where the tissue obtained with a biopsy is rapidly cooled with a cryostat. The cryostat is an instrument that freezes the tissue sample and then cuts it for microscopic section. A glass slide is then firmly held over the thinly sectioned slice, fixed with methanol which makes the cells stable, and then stained usually with Hematoxylin and Eosin to color the cells pink and blue. The pathologist then reads these slides under a microscope, giving an immediate report of whether or not cancer is present in the biopsy specimen. The frozen section technique has become an invaluable tool to assist the surgeon with intraoperative diagnosis.

Dr. Louis B. Wilson, chief of pathology at the Mayo Clinic in Rochester, Minnesota, is routinely credited with developing the technique of the frozen section in 1905. Dr. William Mayo, one of the founders of the Mayo Clinic (along with his brother Charles Mayo, MD), was once quoted as saying, "I wish you pathologists would find a way to tell us surgeons whether a growth is cancer or not while the patient is still on the table".[4] Dr. Wilson clearly saw this need to evaluate tissue during surgery. For freezing tissues, he used the cold (–29 degrees Celsius) January air of Minnesota. According to Mayo Clinic lore – and indeed, part of the story that was told to me and other recently graduated doctors interviewing for residency at the Mayo Clinic in the early 1990s – Dr. Wilson placed a specimen outside his window for just a few minutes to allow it to freeze. "Eureka! The tissue froze and now could be sectioned!" Beginning in 1895, multiple papers by authors at other institutions had also described techniques for freezing tissue. Rightly or wrongly, these authors and institutions have also claimed credit for its invention.

What mattered to me and to John was that after 10 biopsies, the frozen sections were clear. We could now cut out the ulcer and the surrounding cancer, knowing where it stopped its invasion into normal scalp.

The circular incision around the ulcer was made down to the skull (Figure 6.1). The tumor and surrounding radiated scalp were peeled off the bone. Fortunately, the bone appeared like an eggshell, smooth without erosion or cracks. For now, the brain was healthy, cancer-free. My attention now turned to isolating recipient blood vessels. The two closest, in front of the ear, the superficial temporal artery (STA) and vein (STV), were dissected free from the overlying skin and fat. The STA was relatively large, 1.5 mm in diameter, about the diameter of a piece of spaghetti. The STV was also 1.5 mm, perhaps a good match for one of the small veins called the venae comitantes that routinely travel on either side of the radial artery.

The main venous outflow of a RFFF flap is often designed to include the cephalic vein. This large superficial vein is one of the two main veins of the arm. "Cephalic" is derived from the Latin and Greek for "head", which refers to the upward pathway the vein takes as it travels up the arm back to the heart. The cephalic vein is often quite large, 3–4 mm, the diameter of a piece of macaroni. The STV could be sewn (i.e., anastomosed) into the cephalic vein of the RFFF, but such a large mismatch in diameters could place the anastomosis at risk for clotting. The veins in the neck are much bigger, and thus would provide a better size match. "Hold your breath and bear down". With this simple command done before surgery in clinic, I had seen the outline of John's external jugular (EJ) vein bulge in his lateral neck and declare its size. It would be a good size match for the cephalic vein. Therefore, a second incision was made, a 2-cm incision over the shadow of the EJ in the neck. With dissecting scissors, the fat and the thin platysma muscle over the EJ were pushed aside. The EJ, now fully visible, was ready to be sewn to the cephalic vein of the free flap.

Before the widespread use of the anterolateral thigh (ALT) free flap, the RFFF, first performed in 1979 by Chinese surgeon Guofan Yanget,[5] was the workhorse flap for head and neck reconstruction. It is thinner than an ALT flap because a forearm is often less fatty than a thigh. It also has a long pedicle that can reach the neck even when used for cephalic defects, such as those on top of the head. However, once it is raised, the flexor tendons are exposed without the covering of the skin and fat, and the sensory nerve (i.e., the superficial radial nerve) to the back of the thumb and the webspace between the thumb and index finger is at risk. To replace the tissue removed by free flap, skin grafts from the leg are placed over the exposed tendons and nerves of the forearm. Loss or delayed healing of these skin grafts can cause hand stiffness or numbness. Few patients report any significant change in the range of movement, strength, or feeling of their wrist or fingers. However, in patients who depend on their hands for their living (i.e., manual laborers) or enjoyment (i.e., musicians) the RFFF often becomes a secondary option for reconstruction.

John's RFFF was raised without difficulty. The superficial radial sensory nerve was carefully dissected out of the fat and skin of the flap. This takes time and a careful observation and preservation of the small nerve branches going to the thumb and the surrounding skin. Any seemingly small mishandling of the nerve could create a handicap, areas of permanent numbness around the thumb. Quality of life (QOL), not just cancer control, is a desired outcome for any operation. Small mishaps can worsen overall QOL.

QOL typically refers to functional outcome. Any loss of function can become a daily reminder to a patient of their affliction and treatment. From one person to the next, what quality of life means can be entirely different. A critical consideration necessitates a more personal connection with your patients to understand what QOL means. For John, this was his golf game. Golf was more than just a hobby. It was a connection to others and most importantly to his son Tripp, who shared a mutual love of the game. It served as a bedrock for their relationship.

The RFFF was divided from the arm and transferred to the scalp (Figure 6.1). The radial artery and one of its venae comitantes were respectively anastomosed to the STA and STV. The cephalic vein from the flap was tunneled down to the neck for a second venous anastomosis to the EJ vein. After 10 hours of operating, John arrived in the Intensive Care Unit. The ulcer and cancer were now replaced with the normal skin and tissue from the right forearm.

Six weeks later during outpatient follow-up in clinic, with a smile on his face, John told me how he was doing: "I've never seen a better day!". His tumor was gone. No open wound, no pain. Permission to start playing golf was gladly given. John joked: "I think my golf handicap has improved".

Whether it was a new skin cancer or a recurrence, it was impossible to know. Ten months after surgery, a small shallow ulcer erupted on the scalp just at the junction of the healed RFFF with the skin by the left ear. A biopsy showed squamous cell cancer. Surgeons refer to tissue that is known to have an extremely high risk of new cancer as being "condemned". John's "condemned scalp" declared itself and sentenced him to a trial of chemotherapy. The hope was that the cocktail of drugs would slow the tumor growth and delay the occurrence of any additional cancer. Part of his chemotherapy included cetuximab, a targeted cancer drug that is a monoclonal antibody that binds with a protein, called an epidermal growth factor receptor (EGFR), on tumor cells. Cetuximab has shown promising effectiveness against squamous cell carcinoma of the skin, as well as of the oral cavity and pharynx. Somehow, the side effects of the chemotherapy, including nausea, fatigue, and a relentless nagging itch from an ever-present rash, did not distract John from his optimism. Every day was still the best day. The chemotherapy held the cancer at bay for the next 6 months.

It was during these treatments that John and I first began to talk about the hopes for his family, particularly for his youngest son, Connor. Studying business as his major, Connor planned to pursue a line of work in finance, similar perhaps to his father's. John confided that he thought medicine, not finance, might be Connor's passion. Caring for his dad through multiple transplants and related surgeries, Connor had experienced miraculous treatments firsthand. He had also seen the suffering caused by disease and the limitations of medicine. He had spent the time reading the proposed mechanisms and safety profiles of the drugs that his father was prescribed. Acting as the de facto medical liaison between the numerous transplant specialists, surgeons, and intensivists caring for his dad, Connor guided his family through the various medical options and surgical details that were being presented and updated. Without dwelling on the prognosis, John, his family, and I realized that his cancer might not be curable. If I could help Connor in any way to pursue medicine, I assured John that I would.

Seventeen months after his free flap, John prepared for his second scalp resection and flap. The ulcer had grown and was causing relentless pain. This next operation was not easy. Frozen sections around the ulcer were checked, and a wide piece of the surrounding scalp and half of the RFFF were removed. The closest vessels to the defect had already been used for the first free flap. Vein grafts could be harvested, sewn into a branch of the carotid artery or internal jugular vein in the neck, and tunneled to the scalp to place a blood supply near the defect, but additional anastomoses also can present additional opportunities for failure – additional sites that could clot or kink. Perhaps the radial artery and cephalic vein of the previously inset RFFF could be used as the main inflow and outflow to the second flap (Figure 6.2).

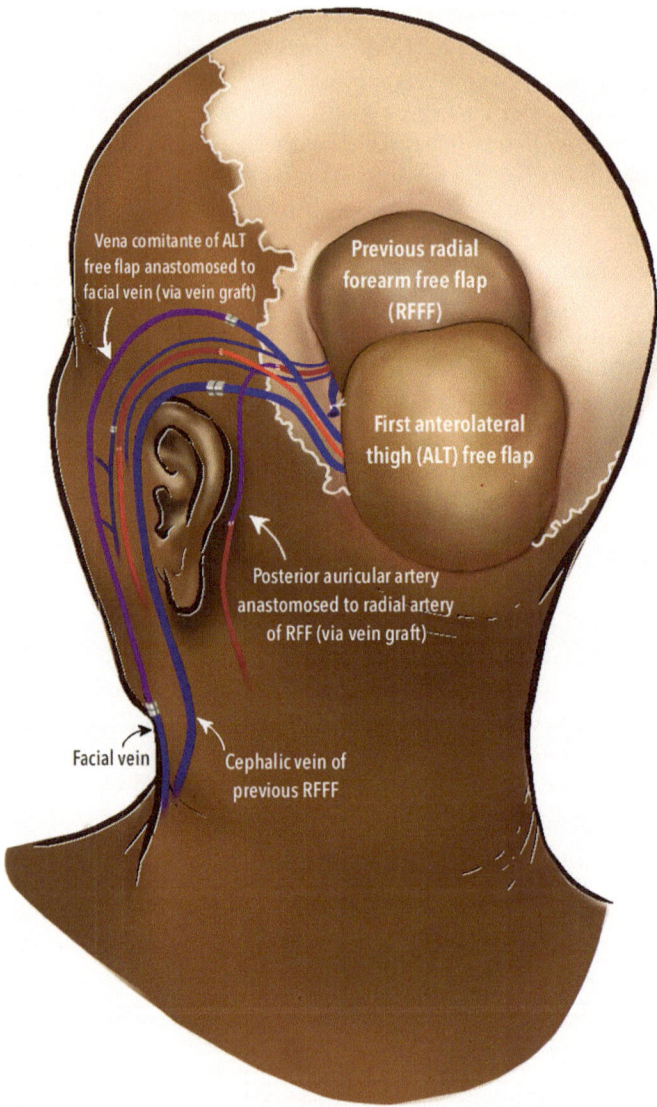

Figure 6.2 The second major operation with an anterolateral thigh (ALT) free flap sewn into a partially resected radial forearm free flap (RFFF).

A larger section of the scalp and the first flap are resected to treat a recurrence of the skin cancer. Multiple vein grafts and additional blood vessels in the neck and behind the ear are used to provide circulation to the second free flap and to the remaining portion of the first free flap.

With a few spreads of my scissors, the radial artery and the cephalic vein proximal to the resection were cleared of the surrounding tissue. They were open, bleeding, and away from the site of the recurrent cancer; they could be used again for additional microsurgery. A vein graft was harvested from the lower leg. It was sewn into a facial vein just above the mandible and tunneled through the face to the scalp so that it could be sewn into the second vena comitante of the ALT free flap. This provided a second venous outflow for the ALT, just in case the first anastomosis to the previously used cephalic vein clotted.

The ALT flap sprung to life with the anastomoses completed. Fresh red blood oozed from the flap edges, and a pulse could be heard across the room with a doppler. However, the part of the RFFF, remaining above where the cancer had been resected, was pale, with only slight bleeding from its cut edges. The cancer resection had divided the mid-portion of the radial artery which had been primarily perfusing this portion of the RFFF. It might be okay. There was some blood supply which was now present from the vascular ingrowth from the surrounding scalp. However, this was random blood supply, not pedicled blood supply. With surgery, you do not leave outcome to chance; you do not just hope it will be okay. You fix it.

Behind the ear, there is a small artery called the post-auricular artery (PAA). The skin here had been partially removed with the cancer resection. Stare at any living piece of flesh stripped of its skin, and you can often see the beat of an artery beneath the fat. Then take a doppler, and gently press it against the exposed tissue to confirm its presence, to hear it beat. The PAA behind John's left ear could indeed be seen and heard. The PAA could be used to restore a pedicled blood supply to the remaining RFFF, but it was 2 inches away from the cut end of the radial artery. Therefore, a second vein graft was harvested from John's thigh. The microscope was positioned over the ear, and with 10x magnification, the vein graft was sewn first to the PAA. With blood pulsing through the vein graft from the PAA, the divided end of the radial artery was then sewn into the vein graft. Perfusion was now restored to the remaining tissue of the RFFF. At 8:17 p.m., 12 hours after we began, John's second major reconstruction was concluded (Figure 6.2).

Six days after surgery, John was discharged from the hospital. His flaps were well perfused, healing. Importantly, his pain was well controlled, nearly gone.

It was during the next few months, as John recovered, that he began to focus his energy on answering how he could help improve the lives, especially of children, undergoing reconstructive surgery. John and I had spoken a number of times about how I routinely performed pediatric microsurgery for children born without the ability to smile, as well as for children with facial tumors and deformities caused by trauma or congenital deformities. Nationally, there are some children's hospitals that can provide these operations. However, some children do not receive this care because of a lack of awareness of the surgical possibilities or a lack of surgeons willing or able to do these operations. Some families with the financial means choose to travel to one of the select few centers in the United States or Canada that provide this care. In contrast, many lower-income pediatric patients do not have this option.

For pediatric patients in Colorado, we could address this inequity. Philanthropic investments would help consolidate efforts to make pediatric microvascular surgery a prioritized surgical sub-specialty. Importantly, funding allowing for a dedicated center would be used to coordinate and enroll clinical services that would comprehensively help children with severe facial deformities. For example, after facial reanimation surgery (i.e., transferring a muscle to restore the ability to smile; see Figure 2.3), physical therapy could provide exercises and instruction to teach children how to smile with minimal effort. To help with any issues of psychological well-being, such as depression and low self-esteem, children could be routinely offered formal psychotherapy. However, both of these services require funding. Pediatric microsurgery and other related services have often been overlooked and under-supported at most academic institutions. This is primarily due to relatively low surgical volumes compared to adult microsurgery, a deficiency of highly trained medical providers, and the extremely low reimbursement rates from Medicaid, often the primary insurance provider for many children.

To John, this cause was personal. He knew these children were undergoing the very same operations that he had endured. Being in finance, John also understood the business aspect of medicine. Our conversations turned to other aspects of plastic surgery care that were struggling due to poor financial support.

For nearly 15 years I had been travelling to Guatemala to perform cleft surgery and burn reconstruction, but during the last 4 years I had changed the focus of these trips to help children born with microtia (Figure 6.3). Microtia is a birth defect that causes a malformed or underdeveloped ear, occurring in approximately 2 to 3 cases per 10,000 live births. To our knowledge, we had established the only routine, annual surgical mission trip to Guatemala, indeed to Central America, which focused on microtia and provided long-term follow-up. Unlike cleft surgery, there is zero to very little capability of providing local surgical care to children with microtia in Guatemala. More than 50% of the population of Guatemala lives below the poverty line, and according to the World Bank, Guatemala has the fourth-highest rate of chronic malnutrition in the world and the highest in Latin American and Caribbean.

This comprehensive and long-term care was possible only by partnering with The Shalom Foundation.[6] In the late 1990s, Steve Moore, former President of the Country Music Association, founded the Shalom Foundation with the vision of "providing critical medical and nutritional care to underprivileged children in Guatemala". The mission of the Shalom Foundation

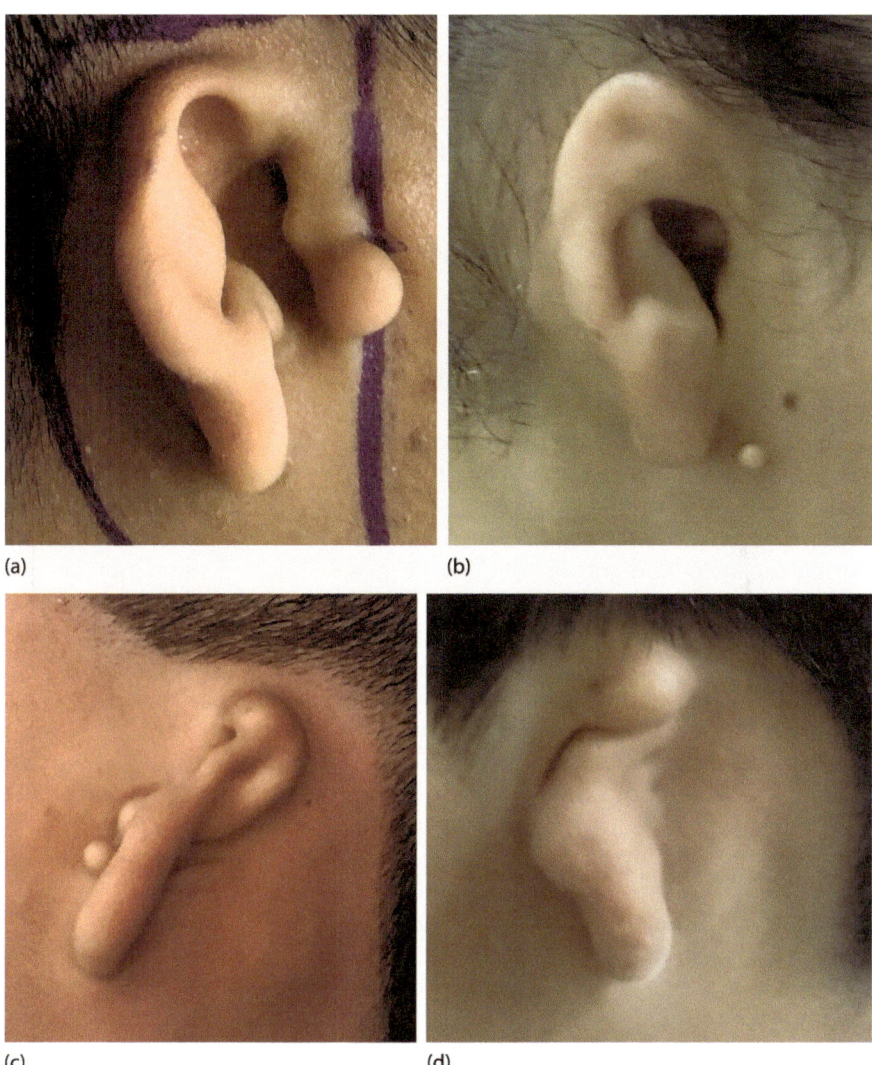

(a)   (b)

(c)   (d)

Figure 6.3 a–d Range of congenital ear anomalies treated during plastic surgery mission trips (supported by the John Lester Foundation) at the Moore Surgical Center in Guatemala.

Microtia, meaning "little ear", varies in appearance and severity.

became clear after Steve encountered a young girl, Ana, who had been caught in the crossfire of a gang fight and hit with a stray bullet. After flying Ana to the United States to receive care, Steve was faced with the harsh realities that many Guatemalan children experience. The majority lack access to quality medical care.

To help address this problem, Steve founded the Shalom Foundation and proceeded to build and fund the Moore Surgical Center in Guatemala City. The center includes three operating rooms, 20 beds for patients, and an employed administrative staff that screens and maintains long-term contact with the patients and their families. The Moore Center provides and, importantly, pays local surgeons and pediatricians to help with the surgical care and follow-up. We and other visiting surgical teams from the United States provide the surgeons, anesthesiologists, and medical supplies, and also donate funds to the Moore Center to assist in paying their staff and to help with the costs of travel and food for the patients and their families. As of this writing, the Shalom Foundation has hosted over 100 medical teams from the United States, distributed over 105,000 meals to vulnerable families, and performed over 6,500 surgeries.

I discussed with John the mission of the Shalom Foundation, the importance of plastic surgery care in Guatemala, and the financial obstacles of doing surgical mission trips. We also discussed the clinical and genetics research that we had designed to complement the surgical care. Annually during the trips and throughout the year, we collected outcomes on our patients, including quality of life data. To determine if there was a genetic cause of microtia, we also collected saliva and samples of discarded tissue from surgery. This saliva and tissue were then frozen on dry ice and sent back to the United States for analysis. The process for creating these studies had been extensive. Consent forms and protocols for collecting data and maintaining patient confidentiality all had to be approved by the Guatemalan Ministry of Health and the appropriate Institutional Review Boards in the United States. Every document was translated into Spanish, and when confronted with a family that did not speak Spanish, at least two translators were needed – one to translate the indigenous Mayan dialect into Spanish, and another to translate from Spanish into English.

The post-surgery questionnaire was extensive. In addition to simply asking about surgical outcomes, potential complications, and the ability to follow up with doctors in Guatemala after we returned to the United States, we asked more qualitative questions. For example, list the positive and negative changes that you attribute to your surgery. Did the operation (Figures 6.4 and 6.5) improve your self-confidence, improve your interactions with your friends, change the way you dress, (i.e., make it less likely that you try to hide your abnormality), help how you see yourself as being successful, or contribute to your ability to being more employable? Would you recommend or do this operation again?

Philanthropic support would allow additional trips to happen each year and ensure long-term sustainability of the international outreach. Focusing on pediatric microsurgery and microtia, John and I started the preliminary work and plans to help this population. He drew up a vast list of potential donors from his work in finance, wrote down his personal perspective and the parallel impact this could have on the children, even writing in his notes:

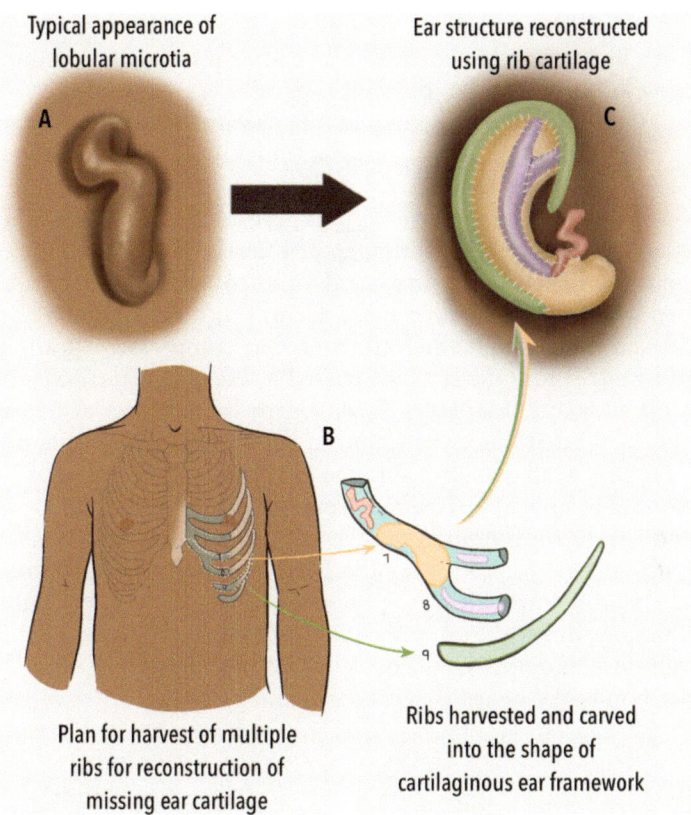

Typical appearance of
lobular microtia

Ear structure reconstructed
using rib cartilage

A

C

B

Plan for harvest of multiple
ribs for reconstruction of
missing ear cartilage

Ribs harvested and carved
into the shape of
cartilaginous ear framework

Figure 6.4 Typical first stage reconstruction of microtia using the patient's ribs.

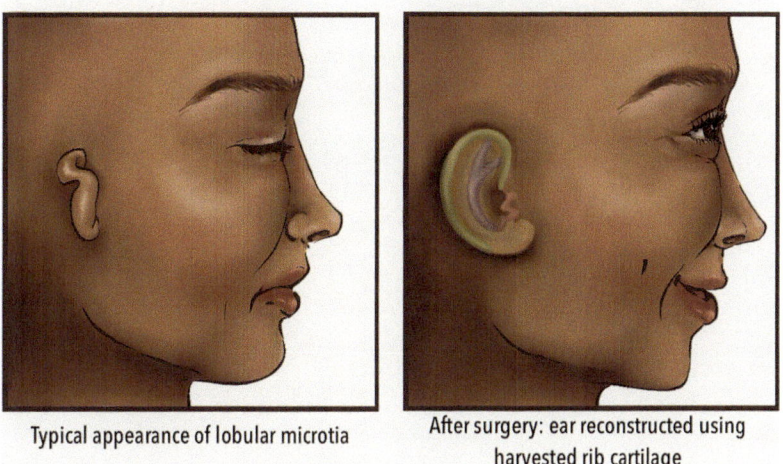

Typical appearance of lobular microtia

After surgery: ear reconstructed using
harvested rib cartilage

Figure 6.5 Typical pre- and postoperative appearance after ear reconstruction.

"This is about allowing children to smile again. It's about giving children new ears. It's about restoring a child's face after a tumor was removed. It's about letting kids get back to their lives again".[7]

As John and I worked on organizing this philanthropic effort to promote the health and QOL of pediatric patients undergoing reconstructive plastic surgery, John once again would battle his own cancer.

The swelling under the flap was not expected. With compression a fluid wave propagated, lifting the flap momentarily as the fluid passed underneath. It was 5 months since his last surgery. The surrounding scalp and the flaps were healed without any ulcer or mass. However, John's pain had returned. He winced and pulled back when the area was compressed. "I am not sure what is going on", I told the family. I passed a needle into the fluid collection and drew off a few milliliters of yellow, slightly brown fluid. A CT scan was ordered. The aspirated fluid was found to have free-floating squamous cancer cells. The CT scan showed that the cortical bone of the skull was no longer smooth but now appeared moth eaten. Moreover, the dura matter, the outer covering (i.e., the outer meninge) of the brain, likely had cancer spreading along it (Figure 6.6). For 2 months John tolerated serial aspirations and additional chemotherapy. However, the pain eventually become unbearable. On a Wednesday, directly from my clinic, John was admitted to the hospital so that high-dose narcotics could be delivered to relieve his pain.

With the family the neurosurgical team and I reviewed the scans and the extent of the cancer. Technically, this could be resected, but should it?

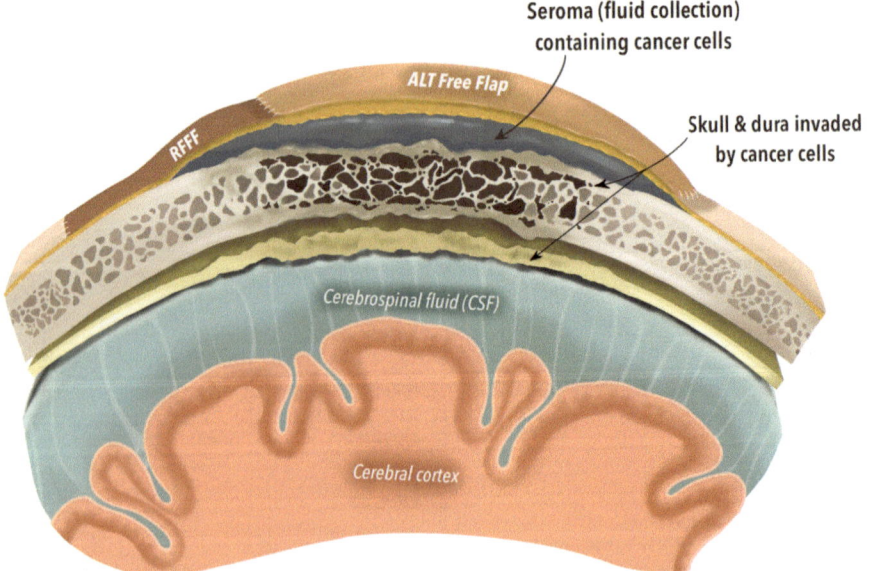

Figure 6.6 Cross section of surgical site showing the recurrent cancer invading skull and dura.

The previous two free flaps would need to be removed in order to expose the underlying skull and dura. Using a bone saw, a large circle cap of bone would be lifted off, and the dura and attached cancer would then be resected. The brain would be fully exposed, with no soft or hard covering. Reconstruction would then be needed to replace everything that was missing.

Cerebrospinal spinal fluid (CSF) is the fluid that surrounds the brain and spinal cord. It provides nourishment, waste removal, and protection for the brain. It is an ultrafiltrate of plasma, the fluid of whole blood. When it leaks, when it is not contained in the sterile environment provided by intact dura and bone, the brain will sink down in the skull, putting pressure on the lower parts of the brain. This can lead to seizures, headaches, nausea, vomiting, and mental status change. If the CSF is exposed to bacteria, it can become infected, leading to meningitis. Without a successful reconstruction, all of this would happen to John.

We outlined the plan for reconstruction to the family. First, the resected dura would be patched with a dural graft manufactured from bovine pericardium. Pericardium is a tough double-layer membrane that surrounds the heart in mammals. It is harvested from bovines (from the Latin for "cow"), cleaned, and processed as a biomaterial that can then be transplanted into humans as a flexible, watertight sheet. This would be sewn to John's cut dural edges as the first layer protecting the brain and preventing a CSF leak. On top of this, the bone of the skull would be replaced with a PolyEtherEtherKetone (PEEK) implant. PEEK is a synthetic, biocompatible polymer (i.e., a material composed of repeating molecular subunits/molecules) that can be manufactured in a commercial lab. There has been no evidence demonstrating any potential carcinogenic or cytotoxic effects of PEEK implants. In the preoperative planning, John's head CT scan would be imported into a 3D scanner. The 3D printer would then print a PEEK implant to exactly match the area of bone that was to be resected. The custom PEEK implant would be delivered, and then on the day of surgery, it would replace the resected bone. The final step, my role, would be to provide the third layer of protection on the brain. The PEEK implant would be covered with a massive free flap.

There are no pain receptors on the brain itself. This feature explains why neurosurgeons can operate on brain tissue without causing discomfort and can even perform some neurosurgical procedures while a patient is awake. The meninges, periosteum (the covering on the bones), and scalp all have pain receptors. If we resected these, hopefully we could alleviate John's pain. However, death, CSF leak, meningitis, flap failure, and brain injury were real possibilities of the operation that we presented. John's response: "Do it, I cannot live with this pain!"

The value of pain relief cannot be overstated. In the 1990s, researchers at the University of Washington (UW) had extensively surveyed head and neck cancer patients before and after surgery with the UW Quality of Life Questionnaire. The one domain that consistently improved after surgery was pain. One study, for which I collected the data and summarized the results, showed that 67% of the patients reported pain relief after extensive surgery to remove their cancer.[8] This relief continued to be present at the last follow-up one year after surgery. For patients who received radiation therapy, only 29% in this nonsurgical group reported pain relief. Pain relief from cancer is an achievable outcome with surgery. It should be considered even if cure is not possible. As a surgeon, you do your best to present an educated guess of the probability that your operation will provide relief. Unfortunately, there is no certainty, especially if the cancer returns.

The day of an operation should be joyous. It is an opportunity to improve someone's life and restore health. On the day of John's third major operation, anxiety – my anxiety – was the overriding emotion. John was no longer just a patient. He was a friend. However, your emotions cannot bubble up to the surface. They will interfere with your ability to be a technician, to make a balanced medical decision, to communicate to the family and to the operating room staff who are counting on you to deliver. You take a deep breath, focus, and put your blinders on. All distractions must be minimized.

Removing the scalp, skull, and dura would be relatively straightforward, but once everything was gone and I was staring at an exposed brain, my reconstruction must work, or John would die. On that day, all that mattered was that I technically perform, that I successfully protected his exposed brain and returned him to his family. Breathe, focus, put your blinders on.

The cerebral hemispheres are the most prominent structures of the brain. The dura is folded in the midline to form the falx cerebri, which separates and descends vertically between the two cerebral hemispheres. Superiorly, the falx cerebri attaches to the superior sagittal sinus, which in essence is a large vein draining the cortex and returning the CSF fluid to the venous system. The outer structure, the cerebral cortex, is highly convoluted, with deep furrows and elevated folds. This allows for the packing of a greater surface area into a small space. John's cerebral cortex looked clean. With the dura removed, no additional cancer could be seen with the naked eye. Some thickening of the dura was present near the sagittal sinus: impossible to resect due to its proximity to the sinus. Previous radiation therapy had made the tissue fibrotic and stiff. We hoped this penny-sized area of thickening was just the typical reaction caused by radiation.

Neurosurgery was done. I began.

With a surgical marker, I outlined the ALT flap that I would harvest from John's right leg. The overall size of an ALT flap is dependent on the number and location of the perforators. What remains uncertain is the maximum dimensions of an ALT free flap that can be harvested based on a single perforator (i.e., a routine ALT free flap). In 2014, we had published in *Plastic and Reconstructive Surgery Global Open* the options and indications for "supercharging and venous augmenting" an ALT free flap.[9] When confronted with extensive head and neck defect, one must determine whether a routine ALT free flap will have sufficient blood flow.[9,10] "Supercharging and venous augmenting" is a technique that involves harvesting a second pedicle

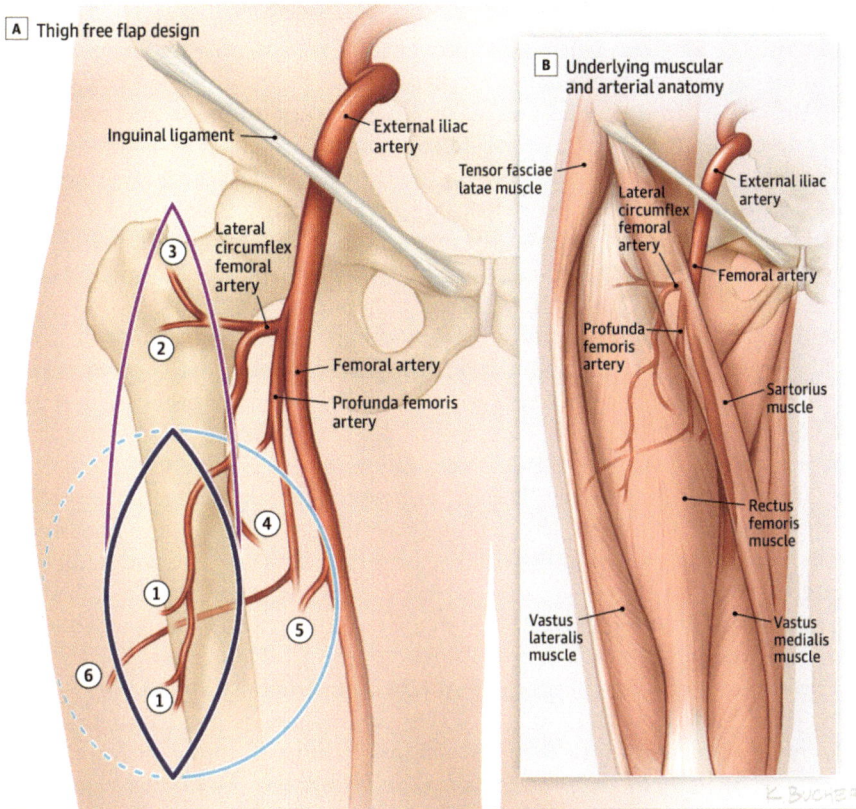

Figure 6.7 Options on how to increase blood flow to thigh free flaps.

Thigh Free Flap Design: Labeled pedicles are the same for main figure and inset. A, possible skin islands; the inset shows underlying musculature and vascular anatomy. The solid dark-blue line indicates a standard ALT flap based off perforator from 1, descending branch of LCFA. The solid purple line indicates an extremely long flap (greater than 17-cm length) based on additional perforator from 2, transverse branch of LCFA or 3, ascending branch of LCFA. The solid light-blue line indicates an extremely wide flap (greater than 12-cm width) based on additional perforator from 4, rectus femoris branch of the descending branch of LCFA or 5, superficial femoral artery. Dashed light-blue line indicates extremely wide flap (greater than 12-cm width) based on additional perforator from 6, profunda femoris. B, Underlying muscular and arterial anatomy. A standard ALT free flap can be supercharged by anastomosing an additional pedicle perfusing perforators 2-5 in the figure. (JAMA Facial Plast Surg, 2018;20(6):468-74.)

with the dominant pedicle (i.e., the descending branch of the lateral circumflex artery and vein) and then connecting this second pedicle, in addition to the dominant pedicle (Figure 6.7). This increases (i.e., augments) the arterial inflow and venous outflow so more flap tissue can reliably be harvested.

By increasing the blood supply, flap complications, in particular partial flap loss, could be avoided. If John had any partial flap loss, the underlying brain could be exposed to the outside world. The defect on John's scalp was massive, the size of an unfolded pocket square. This technique would be a great and reliable solution, but there were some hurdles. All of the nearby vessels in the scalp had been used for the previous two free flaps, and we were running out of vein grafts to extend vascular connections down to the face and neck. I looked at John's right ankle and medial calf. This part of the leg was still healthy, without cancer or scar. I made a mental note: I would go there if I needed another vein graft.

I pressed the Doppler gently across the skin of John's leg. "Whoosh" could be heard at three distinct spots, indicating three distinct perforators perfusing the skin. Importantly, they were separated from each other by 3–4 centimeters and fell along a descending line, indicating that these three perforators originated from the same axial vessels, the descending branch of the lateral circumflex artery (DLCA) and vein. If all three perforators could be dissected into the flap, the massive flap that was being designed would likely have great perfusion. I would not need to harvest a second pedicle.

Indeed, there were three large perforators. They were dissected through the lateral quadricep muscle, the vastus lateralis muscle. Once I reached the origin of the DLCA from the profundus artery, the dissection stopped and the final skin incision around the flap was completed. All of the edges of the flap were bleeding, with no concern that perfusion was decreased along the margins. A 2-cm stump of the STA just above the zygomatic arch remained where the pedicles of the previous flaps had been, but the nearby veins were cauterized or tied off – unusable for microsurgery. The vascular clamp on the STA stump was temporarily released. Blood shot across the surgical drapes. An incision was made in front of the right medial ankle extending up the leg, and 30 centimeters of the greater saphenous vein were harvested. It was cut into two separate vein grafts, sewn into two branches of the jugular venous system in the neck, and then tunneled underneath the skin to the scalp.

With all of the blood supply positioned and flowing, the ALT flap was now divided from the leg and brought to the scalp for the microsurgery. The pedicle of the ALT flap (the DLCA and its two veins) was positioned next to the STA and the two vein grafts. With the vessels and vein grafts magnified by the microscope, they were then sewn together. Twenty hours from the start of the case, after four shifts of anesthesiologists and nurses, we returned John to the ICU and to his family. All detectable cancer was resected; his third flap safely and securely wrapped the brain (Figure 6.8).

John was discharged from the hospital 8 days after the surgery. The resection and reconstruction turned the pain off, or nearly so. Small amounts of pain pills were still necessary, but the pain was easily managed without causing any interference with daily activities or thought. He returned home to his family and part-time work at UBS. An MRI scan 3 months after surgery

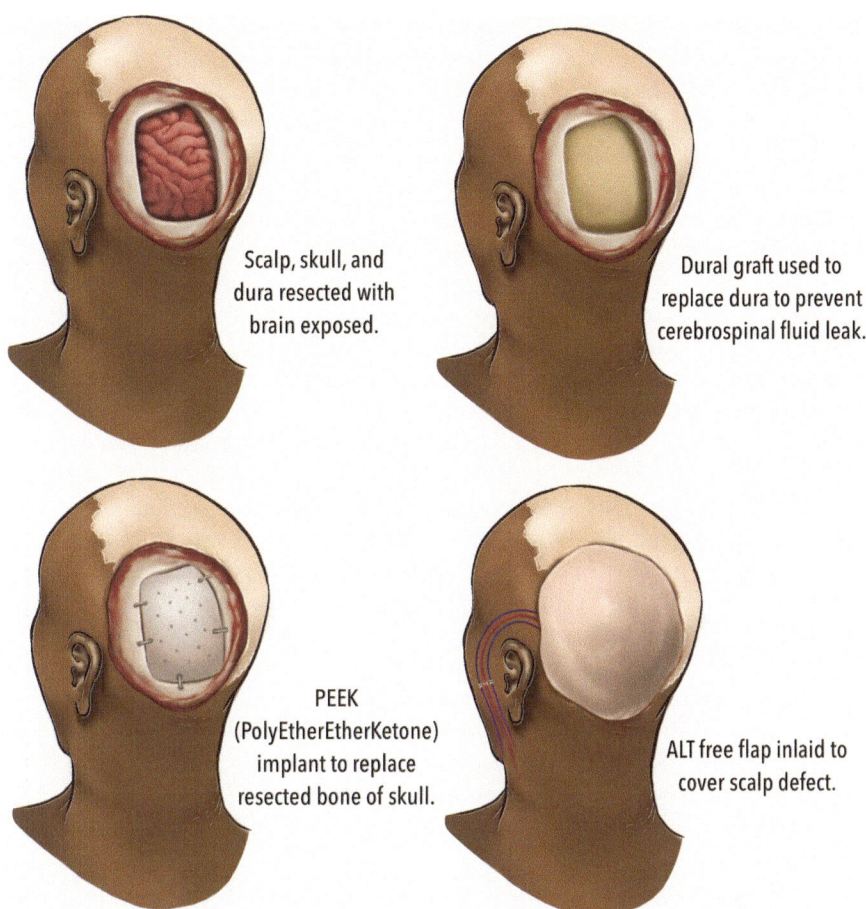

Scalp, skull, and dura resected with brain exposed.

Dural graft used to replace dura to prevent cerebrospinal fluid leak.

PEEK (PolyEtherEtherKetone) implant to replace resected bone of skull.

ALT free flap inlaid to cover scalp defect.

Figure 6.8 The third operation resecting and reconstructing scalp, skull, and dura.

To treat the recurrent cancer the previous 2 free flaps, skull, and dura have been resected. Reconstruction was done with a bovine pericardium to patch the dura, a PEEK implant to replace the bone, and an ALT free flap to replace the resected scalp.

showed no evidence of cancer. For the Christmas break, the family enjoyed a well-deserved holiday vacation in Hawaii.

John, his family, and I all knew that the surgery was likely palliative, not curative. Quality of life, pain relief, and time with his family had been restored. However, a new ulcer, a new cancer, did again present. A small ulcer within the radiated scalp became progressively larger over the next 4 months. CSF fluid began to leak through the wound, and it became infected, leading to meningitis and intractable seizures. Seven months after his third free flap, John underwent one last major operation. The ulcer and additional scalp were resected and replaced with a fourth free flap, his left latissimus muscle.

This sealed the CSF leak and stopped the seizures. John was able to regain strength and some normalcy. He returned home to his family. For an additional 16 months he remained without seizures and relatively pain free.

The cancer, though, was still present below the reconstructed skull, below the PEEK implant on top of the brain, impossible to resect or treat with additional radiation or chemotherapy. Eventually, after 4 years of amazing resilience, John's body, but not his spirit, was finally consumed by his cancer. Surrounded by his family, John C. Lester Jr., my friend, passed on August 30, 2016.

Disease, reconstruction, and recovery are a continuum of suffering and reidentification. Our patients are forever changed even in the best of circumstances. With the surgery complete, the postoperative course uncomplicated, it is easy to feel our job as a surgeon is done.

Yet for the patient and their families, the work never ends; it is an ever-present reality and effort to redefine normal. A periodic clinic visit serves as the only glimpse into this experience and the responsibility we harbor as stewards of post-surgical life. Reconstructive surgery not only represents a surgical solution for the patient, but generates a ripple effect of reidentification, suffering, and support that affects not just the patient and their family, but also their community and colleagues.

John's funeral and celebration of his life were attended by hundreds. Family, college friends, past Denver Broncos, Denver's business leaders, and friends crowed into the packed church. Each told stories of how John had positively impacted their lives through caring for them and their families in times of need. The service was emotional and tearful. How did a man so burdened by his own illness find the energy and will to step out beyond himself?

Connor, fighting back his own tears, told the congregation how his father's optimism and hope for the future always overshadowed his terrible illness. As someone caught in that ripple effect, Connor laid out a vision to leave a lasting legacy for his father – by starting a nonprofit foundation called the John Lester Foundation. It was their hope that they would be able to alleviate the suffering of children and others so that they would have hope and confidence to face their own future.

John's spirit and legacy have thrived. After quitting his job in business, Connor spent the better part of two years fundraising for the John Lester Foundation, assembling a board of his closest friends and family. As of this writing, the foundation has raised over $750,000 for pediatric reconstructive surgery. The John Lester Foundation has grown into a robust organization that is fully funded into the foreseeable future. His family, including his mother and wife, help run the administrative side of the foundation and participate in the annual mission trips to Guatemala, translating, collecting quality of life data, and just being there for families, showing that they care.

Connor's calling became clear. Graduating in 2023 from Georgetown Medical School, Connor was chosen by his graduating medical school class to give the 2023 commencement address. I could hear some of his advice and wisdom originating from his father's character. They are worth repeating:

> We may never know the impact that we have. … As patients and families come and go, we will do our daily job, maybe a little sleep deprived and tired. But no matter what, we will leave a lasting impact, that impact has the power to change lives. So let's carry that responsibility and privilege into the most mundane tasks because in those moments we can make a difference.

Mr John C. Lester has made the day better, not just today, but every future day.

REFERENCES

1. Dychtwald K. *Radical curiosity: one man's search for cosmic magic and a purposeful life*. The Unnamed Press, April 6, 2021.
2. https://agewave.com/live-your-legacy/
3. Executive Edge: John Lester, June 22, 2009. https://www.coloradobiz.com/
4. Gal AA. The centennial anniversary of the frozen section technique at the Mayo Clinic. *Arch Pathol Lab Med* (2005);129(12):1532–1535.
5. Hongyi W, Guo B, Hui Q, Jiang D, Liu X, Tao K. The first case of free radial forearm skin flap: a 40-year follow-up study. *Chinese Journal of Plastic and Reconstructive Surgery* 2020;2(3):177–180.
6. https://www.theshalomfoundation.org
7. https://www.johnlesterfoundation.org
8. Deleyiannis FWB, Weymuller EA, Coltrera MD. Quality of life of disease-free survivors of advanced (Stage III or IV) oropharyngeal cancer. *Head Neck* 1997 Sept;19(6):3466–3473.
9. Deleyiannis FWB, Badeau AM, Leem TH, Song JI. Supercharging and augmenting venous drainage of an anterolateral thigh free flap: options and indications. *Plast Reconstr Surg Glob Open* 2014 May 7;2(4):e135.
10. King BBT, Rodriguez IE, Deleyiannis FWB. Indications and outcomes of single-pedicle vs 2-pedicle thigh free flaps in head and neck reconstruction. *JAMA Facial Plast Surg*, 2018;20(6):468–474.

Chapter 7

Value, options, and cost of clinical research

Research is formalized curiosity. It is poking and prying with a purpose.
– Zora Neale Hurston, 1891–1960
American author and anthropologist

"Dr. D, your patient is smoking in the preop area!", the charge nurse exclaimed. Indeed, she was, but all I could see was the patient sucking on a small metal tube and some vapor being emitted, no smoke. My teenage patient, a 16-year-old with a dollar-sized piece of her scalp missing, was casually smoking an electronic cigarette (e-cigarette) just outside the operating room. She was scheduled today for an ALT free flap to reconstruct her scalp. "Do you want to cancel the case?", the nurse asked. It was 2013, and this was the first time I had ever seen an e-cigarette. I had never considered how it could affect a surgical outcome.

As a surgeon, you hope to control all things, either real or perceived, that could affect your patient. Blood loss, staff that work on your team, your own medical preparedness, time of your case, even the hours you sleep the night before the case, you try to control so that your patient does the best. You cannot control the detrimental effects of lifestyle or some of the illnesses (i.e., comorbidities) that patients bring with them. Smoking, obesity, diabetes, and cardiovascular disease are just a few of these patient factors. Taking these comorbidities into consideration, you learn as a surgeon how to modify your operation to give a patient the best chance of success. You learn when to refuse to do an operation and when to wait so that any patient factors, such as smoking, diabetes, or obesity, can be better managed prior to surgery.

This learning begins with learning basic physiology as a student, continues with reviewing published articles that you relate and extrapolate to your own patients, and culminates in critically analyzing your own results and publishing these so that others can learn from them. This final step is the real challenge. It takes time away from actually seeing patients, involves no financial reward, and potentially exposes you to criticism if your published results are not up to "the standard". However, it also makes you really

DOI: 10.1201/9781003538028-8

think. It makes you better by questioning assumptions and pushes you to prove to yourself that your treatment is the right plan.

Eldora is a wind-swept ski slope outside Boulder, Colorado. It is a great place for young kids to learn how to ski. Avoiding the cold, the adults tend to congregate inside the gym-like waiting room, drinking coffee and reading while their children ski or take lessons. On February 22, 2014, as I tried to entertain myself while I waited for my daughters, the Health section of *The New York Times* caught my eye. An article entitled "The New Smoke – A Hot Debate over E-Cigarettes as a Path to Tobacco, or from It" by Sabrina Tavernise announced the idea that e-cigarettes might be considered a disruptive innovation.[1]

Sales of electronic cigarettes had more than doubled from 2012 to 2013, totaling $1.7 billion. The use of e-cigarettes had been surging in popularity, potentially because they were viewed as a healthier alternative to tobacco cigarettes. Health experts like to say that people smoke for the nicotine but die from the tar. E-cigarettes took the deadly tar out of the equation while offering the nicotine fix and the sensation of smoking. However, there were multiple skeptics to the assumption about the relative health benefits of e-cigarettes. According to the report, Stanton A. Glantz, a professor of medicine at the University of California, San Francisco, was convinced that

> e-cigarettes may erase the hard-won progress achieved over the last half-century in reducing smoking. He predicted that the modern gadgetry will be a glittering gateway to the deadly, old-fashioned habit for children, and that adult smokers will stay hooked longer now that they can get a nicotine fix at their desks.[1]

It was obvious from the article that the popularity of e-cigarettes was outpacing the knowledge concerning their safety. In regard to surgical safety, in particular to plastic surgery outcomes, in 2014 there were absolutely no data. In fact, one might assume that surgical complications might increase due the increasing demand and the resultant increased consumption of nicotine.

The harmful effects of smoking tobacco are relatively well described. Tobacco smoke, due to its nicotine content and to its non-nicotine particulates (i.e., tar), has a deleterious effect on the cardiovascular system, angiogenesis (i.e., blood vessel formation) and skin capillary perfusion. Specifically, it has been shown to damage the endothelium (i.e., the cells lining the inside of arteries and veins) and impair endothelium-dependent vasorelaxation. The damaged endothelium subsequently activates platelets, which release the potent vasoconstrictor thromboxane A_2, further inducing vasoconstriction and thrombogenesis (i.e., formation of small clots in capillaries). This effect persists even after abstaining from smoking in chronic smokers. This constriction and damage of blood vessels combined with clots chokes blood supply, which leads to the poor perfusion of tissue. This in turn can cause the tissue to die.

Nicotine is frequently identified as the main agent within tobacco smoke that causes these detrimental cardiovascular effects. It is a stimulant drug, but also a toxin that amplifies the platelet-activating, endothelium-damaging, and vasoconstrictive effects of tobacco smoke, resulting in the reduction of tissue perfusion. Nicotine also contributes to tissue hypoxia (i.e., decreased supply of oxygen) by inhibiting prostaglandin I_2, a potent vasodilator and inhibitor of platelet aggregation. Not only do the vessels remain constricted, but the increased platelet aggregation leads to capillary occlusion and further hypoxia. Just as a smoker can easily become short of breath, a smoker's tissue becomes starved of oxygen. All of these effects can cause necrosis of skin, especially if the skin is raised, surgically manipulated, as done in raising a flap.

Knowing that tobacco smoke and nicotine use puts all skin flaps at a significant risk of tissue necrosis, plastic surgeons routinely will not perform elective procedures that involve the raising of a skin flap on patients who smoke. Facelifts, breast reductions, breast lifts, and/or tummy tucks are likely to be denied to patients who smoke until they have quit smoking for at least a month. The risk of a poor surgical outcome is simply too great. Smoking can also decrease perfusion to free and pedicled flaps, but the blood supply to these flaps is often so robust that skin loss and poor wound healing may not occur as often compared to skin flaps with just a random (i.e., subdermal) blood supply. As a result, in contrast to patients undergoing an elective procedure, patients with an acute problem caused by cancer or trauma will still often be offered reconstruction with a free flap even if they are active smokers. The benefit of the flap reconstruction outweighs the smaller risk of flap necrosis.

The teenager's scalp reconstruction with the ALT free flap went well. When last seen 3 months after surgery, her skull was no longer exposed. The flap had patched the missing scalp. She reached into her pocket to show me the brightly colored blue e-cig container. I asked if she was still smoking. She replied, "No, just these e-cigs. It's not really smoking!".

The Food and Drug Administration started regulating the manufacturers of e-cigarettes only in May 2016. This meant that manufacturers were not required to perform safety testing, nor did they have to list the ingredients within the fluid. In general, e-cigarette liquids (e-liquids) contain five main ingredients: nicotine, water, glycerol, propylene glycol, and optional flavoring. When one inhales, the device heats the e-liquid and transforms it into an inhalable vapor containing nicotine. Even now, consumers do not know the complete risks of e-cigarettes. Until recently, there were no published studies about the long-term effects of inhaling vaporized nicotine, nor was it known whether there are consequences to the sustained ingestion of propylene glycol, the flavoring, or any of the other unlabeled ingredients.

Reading *The New York Times* article in the Eldora Ski Lounge in 2014, it was clear that I was still in no position to offer my young patient, or any future patient, an informed opinion about e-cigarette smoking. Maybe her flap healed well, precisely because she was smoking e-cigarettes instead of tobacco. However, with a little bit of work and planning, I could likely provide some answers.

Clinical research places a critical role in evaluating treatment outcomes. Research is generally considered primary if data are expressly collected to answer a clinical question. Within primary research there are observational and interventional studies. Observational studies are those studies where the investigator is not acting upon the study participants, but instead observes the association between certain factors and outcomes. These are often large epidemiological studies or large case series of patients who have undergone a particular intervention, such as a type of surgery. Any noted difference in outcome or disease is then explained by how patient or treatment factors may differ between groups of patients. Interventional studies, also called experimental studies, are those where the investigator intervenes usually by providing two different treatments to similar groups of patients and then determining whether there is a difference in outcome.

An observational study to determine the effects of e-cigarettes on any aspect of health, including pulmonary function, cardiovascular disease, and/or skin perfusion, would likely take thousands of patients and years of time collecting and analyzing data. Consider the long-term observational study, known as the British Doctors Study (BDS).[2,3] The BDS is considered a milestone in the field of smoking research because it provided the first strong statistical proof of the correlation between smoking habits and many serious diseases, including lung cancer.

Cigarettes went into broad use in the 1920s – and by the 1940s, lung cancer rates had exploded. In the 1950s, more Americans had died from smoking than in all the wars the United States had fought, but there was still no large prospective study that conclusively demonstrated the health risks of smoking.

The work on the BDS by English physician Richard Doll (1912–2005) and English epidemiologists and statisticians Austin Bradford Hill (1897–1991) and Richard Peto (b. 1943) revolutionized our understanding of the detrimental effects of smoking. Remarkably, the study was carried out on a population of doctors, followed up for 50 years. The choice of this cohort was brilliant. In order to work in the United Kingdom, doctors must continually update their names on the British Medical Register. Thus, the doctors could be easily identified and followed. Moreover, the collection of data, concerning cause of death and any health problems, would be easy to verify since this group of subjects would have routine access to high-level medical care. In 1951, Doll and Hill sent the initial questionnaire about smoking habits to all the doctors working in the United Kingdom. They collected 34,440 questionnaires from male doctors who were 35 years of age or older and started long-term follow-up of observing mortality and cause of death. Because there were few women doctors at the time, women were excluded from the study. The follow-up of the cohort continued until 2001, and through the decades new questionnaires were sent to the study subjects (in 1957, 1966, 1971, 1978, 1991, and 2001) in order to gather information on changes in smoking habits and medical history.

After the first 10 years of follow-up, 4,597 doctors had died. In a number of publications, Doll, Hill, and Peto described the associations (increased risks) between smoking and lung cancer, cancers of the upper respiratory and digestive tracts, chronic bronchitis, peripheral vascular disease, and coronary artery disease. The risk of death from lung cancer was related to the amount of tobacco smoked. For example, the annual death rate in men who smoked 35 or more cigarettes per day (3.15 per 1,000) was 45 times higher than the annual death rate of nonsmokers (0.07 per 1,000). Last but not least, the paper on the 50-year follow-up, published in 2004, confirmed the association between smoking habits and vascular disease, multiple cancers, and pulmonary disease. In this last part of the study, the authors also found that men born during the years 1900–1930 who smoked cigarettes continuously died about 10 years younger than lifelong nonsmokers. Stopping smoking at any age was also associated with an improved life expectancy.

Observational studies, like the BDS, may eventually be done to confirm the effects of electronic cigarettes on health. Professional epidemiologists, not busy clinical surgeons, will likely do these studies. However, surgeons can obtain the formal training of an epidemiologist and biostatistician if they so choose. Such an education, even just a collaboration with a clinical epidemiologist, can lead to a remarkably improved understanding of how best to treat your patients.

Residents in the Department of Otolaryngology–Head and Neck Surgery (Oto-HNS) at the University of Washington (UW) in the 1990s were offered the unique opportunity to pursue formal graduate training in the School of Public Health. For 12 months, residents were excused from clinical responsibilities to study epidemiology, biostatistics, and/or health outcomes. "Surgeons should be clinical scientists, not necessarily basic scientists", was the often-repeated advice of Dr. Ernest Weymuller, chairman of the UW Department of Oto-HNS. Indeed, it was the best advice, advice that I have similarly given to medical students and residents over the years. A clear understanding of epidemiology and biostatistics enables you to become a better clinician because you can properly analyze your own data, design your own clinical studies, and critically review any published paper. Surgeons can rarely run a basic science lab unless they significantly decrease their time operating and/or hire a number of PhD scientists or residents in training to actually do the daily work in the laboratory. Surgeons trained with the skills of an epidemiologist can do their own work, with their own patients as their data, without isolating themselves in a laboratory and without necessarily decreasing their clinical work.

The separate focus of clinical epidemiologists versus surgeons can also offer unique opportunities to answer clinical questions. Epidemiologists are typically focused on determining what causes a disease, whereas surgeons are focused on the outcome of treating the disease. To learn how to code, categorize, and then statistically analyze data, students in biostatistics are given problem sets to work through. This work becomes anything but boring when you begin to envision how your own clinical questions could be structured into a data set that could then be analyzed to answer questions about your own patients. In 1994 during my research year as an otolaryngology resident, I spent the majority of my time working with Dr. David B. Thompson, Professor of Epidemiology, at the Fred Hutchinson Cancer Institute in Seattle. It was during this time that I began to realize the value of collaboration with clinical scientists outside the relatively small world of surgery. This became particularly relevant in regard to determining how we could best predict survival in patients with head and neck cancer.

Survival predictions are traditionally based primarily on the TNM (i.e., Tumor Node Metastasis) stage. Patients with large tumors (i.e., advanced T stage) and with tumors that have spread to lymph nodes or distant sites, such as the lung or liver, have a decreased average survival. Stage IV labels a patient as having the worst overall chance of long-term survival. However, within any large group of patients with cancer, we know that some patients with Stage I cancer may die sooner or do worse than a patient with Stage IV cancer. If you as a surgeon can recognize the additional patient factors that may affect survival, then you can better understand prognosis and tailor your treatment recommendation. For example, if you assume that a patient with an advanced cancer (i.e., Stage IV) will die soon no matter what treatment is offered, then you are not going to offer an extensive surgery. However, as stated, not all patients with extensive cancers are going to do poorly. The question remains how to identify, and how to better stratify patients into distinct groups with more selective, patient-specific treatment.

Alvan R. Feinstein, MD, the founding Director of Yale's Robert Wood Johnson Clinical Scholars Program, had a simple message to the Yale medical students to whom he taught the course, Introduction to Clinical Medicine: "Raise the intellectual level of clinical research". The best clinical data are provided by patients. Learn or devise indexes, rating scales, or other expressions to describe symptoms, physical signs, or clinical phenomena. These indexes or scales can then be used to better understand disease, predict prognosis, and guide treatment. In fact, it was Dr. Feinstein who coined the term "comorbidity" to describe those conditions outside the primary diagnosis that could independently affect prognosis and treatment.[4] To this day, I still remember Dr. Feinstein grumbling, somewhat barking to us, "you need to harden the soft clinical research, to make the patient the center of clinical research. Clinical medicine is much more than molecular biology and lab values".

Alcohol consumption has long been recognized as being highly prevalent among patients with head and neck (i.e., mouth and throat) cancer. Despite this recognition, whether or not alcoholism or any features of alcoholism, such as number of drinks per day or abstinence, affects survival once a patient has been diagnosed with a head and neck cancer had not been adequately evaluated up to the 1990s. Clinicians had speculated that alcoholic patients may have a poorer prognosis than nonalcoholic patients because of a more advanced stage of cancer, the immunosuppressive effects of alcohol, and/or an increased rate of death due to other alcohol-related diseases. To answer these questions, one needs a large population-based group of patients who at the time of cancer diagnosis are questioned about alcohol consumption and health problems related to alcohol consumption. Then, these patients, just like the doctors in the BDS, must be followed for years to evaluate how their alcohol use and alcoholism may affect survival.

Fortunately, Dr. David Thomas and his fellow epidemiologists at the Fred Hutchinson Cancer Center in the late 1980s had collected the first part of such a data set to examine the associations between alcoholism and cancer. They sought to determine what factors of alcohol consumption might cause cancer. In their research they had identified through the Surveillance, Epidemiology, and End Results (SEER) Program of the National Cancer Institute (NCI) all patients living in the Seattle metropolitan area that had developed head and neck cancer from September 1983 through February 1987. Then, these patients within a few months of their diagnosis were contacted to conduct an in-person interview, focusing on a detailed history of their alcohol consumption and health problems related to alcohol (such as pancreatitis, liver problems, and/or history of alcohol withdrawal symptoms). The Michigan Alcohol Screening Test (MAST) was also administered to each patient to determine whether a patient would be considered/classified as an alcoholic. Patients were also questioned about any other factor, such as smoking, that could cause cancer. From this data, Dr. Thomas and his colleagues had subsequently published multiple studies detailing how alcoholism places patients at risk for developing cancer and how this risk varied based on where the cancer occurred (i.e., in the mouth/throat versus the larynx versus the esophagus).

In 1994 after discussing with Dr. Thomas the results of his previous epidemiology studies, the wisdom of Dr. Feinstein came rushing back into my mind. Why not use the previously collected data about alcoholism to develop a clinical index of alcoholism to help determine which patients with head and neck cancer might do better or worse than expected? At that time, the TNM stage was the primary indicator, often the only one, that doctors were using to predict prognosis. Moreover, since the data had been collected in the 1980s, long-term survival (i.e., 5-year survival) on all patients could be determined. Fortunately, the SEER Program registries also routinely collect data on patient demographics, TNM stage, first course of treatment, and follow-up for survival and cause of death.

Having just learned how to create databases and run the statistics from my course work, I linked Dr. Thomas's data with the SEER data and began the analysis. The results published in 1996 in the *Journal of the National Cancer Institute* provided new and important prognostic information and treatment recommendations.[5] Alcoholism and a history of alcohol-related liver disease, pancreatitis, delirium tremens, or seizures (e.g., alcohol-related systemic health problems) were associated with more than a doubling of the risk of death, whereas abstinence from alcohol consumption was associated with a decreased risk of death. These associations were independent of age, tumor site, anatomical stage, histopathologic grade, antineoplastic treatment, and smoking. Alcoholics who were abstinent prior to the diagnosis of their tumor and who did not have a history of alcohol-related systemic health problems had an overall 5-year survival estimate nearly identical to that found for nonalcoholics. Alcoholics with a history of alcohol-related systemic health problems had the worst prognosis; however, even for this group of patients, abstinence prior to tumor diagnosis was associated with increased survival.

Perhaps the most important finding of our study was that abstinence from alcohol prior to the diagnosis of cancer was associated with a statistically significant increase in survival. This finding suggested that sobriety among alcoholic patients with head and neck cancer can lead to prolonged survival. In the 1990s, treatment for alcoholism was not a routine part of head and neck cancer therapy. Our study suggested that treatment should focus not just on the cancer, but also on the complete patient. This approach has now become a standard of care. In 2024, alcoholics with head and neck cancer are routinely offered treatment for alcoholism at the time of their diagnosis. Individualized interventions are designed to educate patients about the specific health benefits of abstaining from drinking, to encourage patients to try abstaining again, and to teach behavioral skills that reinforce drinking cessation.

What made our study so impactful was the superb quality of the data collected by the epidemiologists of Dr. Thomas's team. Questionnaires were carefully designed to be reliable and to capture all habits and health problems related to alcohol consumption. Then, over 4 years, these were methodically administered in person or over the phone as each patient was identified in the SEER registry with a new cancer.

An observational study of e-cigarettes with a similar design to our study of alcoholism would be ideal, but such a design faces large obstacles. There may be many patients who smoke e-cigarettes, but there are just a few that are undergoing any type of flap surgery. Moreover, the e-cigarette smoking history, just like a history of alcohol consumption, would have to be carefully questioned and quantified. The surgical outcomes that may be affected by smoking e-cigarettes would also have to be carefully measured. Subtle differences in outcome, such as partial flap necrosis, wound complications, or surgical infections, would need to be carefully measured. These outcomes are much harder to reliably measure compared to more obvious outcomes, such as survival. Any other factor, such as type of flap, surgical technique, and surgeon experience, would also need to be statistically considered. It would take years and the recruitment of numerous, salaried researchers to conduct such a study.

In such a scenario where numerous obstacles may hinder a well-designed observational study, a clinical investigator can instead turn to animal experimental research. To evaluate whether a risk factor, such as smoking, could affect a surgical outcome, one can perform the surgery on the animal and then also expose the animal to the risk that one is evaluating. With a well-designed experimental model, all of the factors that might affect surgical outcomes can potentially be controlled. The investigator can precisely deliver and measure the amount of nicotine, set the duration of smoking and quantity of cigarettes smoked, and design each operation to be exactly the same.

Within the field of tobacco research, a well-established rat model did indeed exist. This model had been used in previous research mainly to evaluate the effects of smoking on the lungs, and a few studies had also used the model to evaluate how smoking tobacco might affect the survival of skin flaps. In these experiments, rats were typically placed in a closed chamber and exposed to the smoke of tobacco for a number of hours each day. A skin flap was then raised on the back on the rat, keeping the blood supply attached at the flap's base but dividing the blood supply from the sides.

Rats would be divided into two groups. All of the rats would have the same flap surgery, but one group would be exposed to tobacco smoke and the other, acting as the control, would not be exposed to smoke. After the flap surgery, usually at about a week, the flaps would be examined to measure what percentage of the tissue was still alive (i.e., without necrosis). Flaps exposed to tobacco smoke routinely show increased flap necrosis compared to flaps not exposed to tobacco smoke. These results gave credibility to surgeons' universal recommendations that smoking should be stopped prior to elective procedures, especially prior to elective cosmetic procedures.

Could a similar experiment be conducted for e-cigarettes? Searching the research profiles of the faculty in the Division of Pulmonology, I found one researcher, Laima Taraseviciene-Stewart, PhD, who had done pulmonary research using smoking chambers at the University of Colorado. A quick Google search also revealed one company in California, Teague Enterprises, that had just developed a smoking chamber specifically designed for e-cigarettes. After a phone call with Teague Enterprises and a few meetings with Dr. Taraseviciene-Stewart, I realized that we indeed could do the experiment. After we wrote a grant proposal, the Department of Surgery awarded $40,000 for the study, and an e-cigarette smoking chamber was subsequently purchased. With the majority of the experimental daily work done by Aline Rau, MD, Becky Trinh, MD, and Ivan Rodriguez, MD (i.e., surgical residents who were spending a year doing research), we began the experiments.

The purpose of the study was to evaluate the toxic effects on microcirculation and perfusion that e-cigarettes may have in comparison with tobacco cigarettes.[6] Fifty-eight rats were randomized to either exposure to room air, tobacco cigarette smoke, medium-nicotine content (1.2%) e-cigarette vapor, or a high-nicotine content (2.4%) e-cigarette vapor. After 4 weeks of exposure, a random pattern, 3 × 9 cm skin flap was elevated on the dorsum of the rats (Figure 7.1). At 5 weeks, flap survival was evaluated quantitatively, and the rats were euthanized. Plasma was collected for nicotine and cotinine

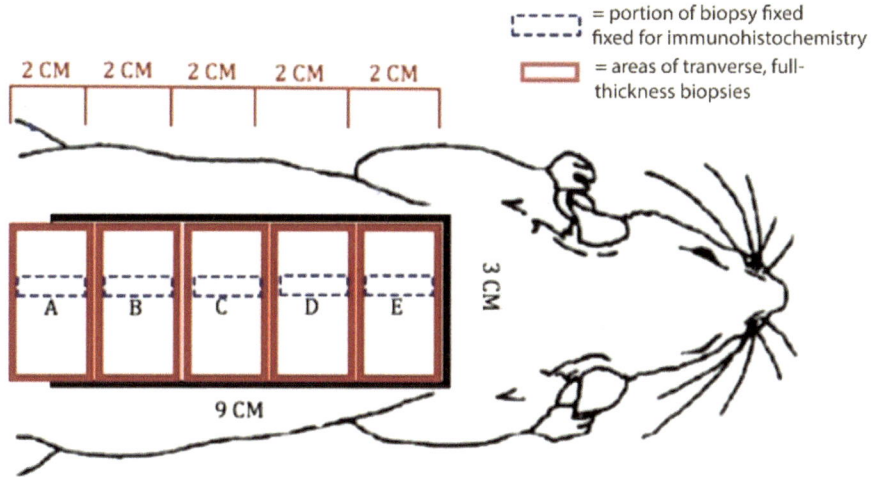

Figure 7.1 Experimental design for evaluating the effects of electronic cigarettes on skin flap necrosis.

Flap harvest – a 9 cm x 3 cm flap was raised on the back of rats. The percentage of flap necrosis was then measured after rats were exposed to the vapor of electronic cigarettes, tobacco smoke, or normal room air. [Reprinted from Electronic cigarettes are as toxic to skin flap survival as tobacco cigarettes (Fig.1, p.88), by Aline Rau, Viktorija Reinikovaite, Eric Schmidt, Laima Taraseviciene-Stewart, Frederic White-Brown Deleyiannis, *Ann Plas Surg*, 2017 (Copyright 2017 by Wolters Kluwer Health, Inc)]

analysis, and flap tissues were harvested for histopathological analysis. Evaluation of the dorsal skin flaps demonstrated significantly increased necrosis in the vapor and tobacco groups (Figure 7.2). The average necrosis within the groups was as follows: control, 19.23%; high-dose vapor, 28.61%; medium-dose vapor, 35.93%; and tobacco cigarette, 30.15%. Although the e-cigarette and tobacco cigarette groups did not differ significantly, each individual group had significantly more necrosis than the control group ($P < 0.05$). These results were corroborated with histopathological analysis of hypoxic tissue.

Both the medium-content and high-nicotine-content e-cigarette exposure groups had similar amounts of flap necrosis and hypoxia when compared with the tobacco cigarette exposure group. These results confirmed that nicotine-containing e-cigarette vapor was similarly toxic to skin flap survival as tobacco cigarettes. We now had the first data from live animals from which surgeons could base their recommendations to patients. Patients should not consider e-cigarettes as a healthy alternative to tobacco smoke. They can cause flap necrosis, just like tobacco cigarettes. Moreover, we followed up this study by then examining the effects of e-cigarettes on the lungs of the rats. E-cigarette vapor was associated with significant ($p < 0.01$) emphysematous lung

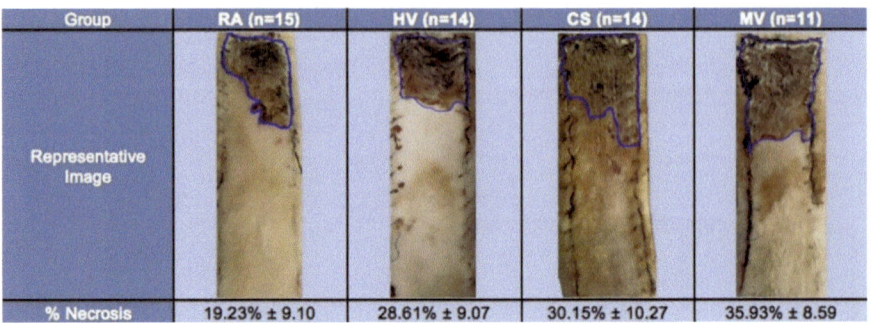

Figure 7.2 Flap necrosis in each experimental group.

RA – Room Air; HV – High Dose Vapor from E-Cigarettes; MV – High Dose Vapor from E-Cigarettes: CS – Cigarette (i.e., Tobacco) Smoke. The darker areas outlined in blue are the areas of the flaps that have died. The vapor from e-cigarettes caused as much necrosis (i.e., death) of the skin flaps as tobacco smoke. [Reprinted from Electronic cigarettes are as toxic to skin flap survival as tobacco cigarettes (Fig.2, p.89), by Aline Rau, Viktorija Reinikovaite, Eric Schmidt, Laima Taraseviciene-Stewart, Frederic White-Brown Deleyiannis, *Ann Plas Surg*, 2017 (Copyright 2017 by Wolters Kluwer Health, Inc)]

destruction when compared to controls (i.e., rats not exposed to vapor). The results were published in 2018 in the *European Respiratory Journal* and provided clinicians additional evidence for their recommendations against smoking e-cigarettes.[7]

Only with sufficient numbers can a surgeon be in position to offer something new, to really determine what factors contribute to good surgical outcomes or to determine what causes disease. Experimental animal surgery is one way to overcome this obstacle. Rats can be purchased, and a large number of surgeries can be done in a relatively short period of time. Otherwise, it often takes a surgeon years of operating to treat enough patients that a complete data set with long-term follow-up can be accrued. This is especially relevant when performing relatively infrequent surgery, evaluating a rare disease, or doing surgery that is more complex and time-consuming. A "research blitz" is one way that these limitations can be overcome.

This concept of a "research blitz" refers to treating a large number of a patients during a short period of time. Surgical mission trips, particularly to underserved countries, present a unique opportunity to evaluate a large number of patients during a short period of time.

Beginning in 2002, I traveled annually to Guatemala with multiple teams to treat children born with birth defects, such as a cleft (i.e., of the lip and/or palate), microtia (i.e., malformed or absent ears), or suffering from burns. In 2004, Dr. Mary L. Marazita, PhD, Professor in the Department of Human Genetics, and Co-Director of the Center for Craniofacial and Dental Genetics at the University of Pittsburgh, reached out to discuss the possibility of expanding their genetic research to the children and their families whom we were evaluating and treating each year in Guatemala. During each surgical mission, which typically lasted one week, hundreds of patients with clefts and their families would present for surgical treatment. In one week we would evaluate more cleft patients than an American cleft team at a university children's hospital would see in a whole year.

The research design involved expanding the phenotype of orofacial clefting.[8] Prior to Dr. Marazita's research, patients were primarily labeled as having a cleft abnormality if there was an obvious cleft of the lip and/or palate. Dr. Marazita wished to explore whether non-overt signs of clefting could be detected and then correlated to genetic markers. The first non-overt sign of clefting on which we would focus were breaks in the muscle, the orbicularis oris, surrounding the upper lip (Figure 7.3). These areas of muscle discontinuity could not be seen with the naked eye but could be detected with an ultrasound (Figure 7.4). The research protocol involved having the entire family of the cleft patient coming to the clinic on the day of the child's cleft surgery. The genetics team would then administer a demographic questionnaire, record a family pedigree, perform an ultrasound of the upper lip (Figure 7.5), and collect a blood sample for DNA analysis from each family member.[9]

Over the next 6 years we collected data from 929 family members and cleft children in Guatemala. In 2004, we also took the cleft "research blitz" to the Hospital Infantil Universitario Nino Jesus in Madrid, Spain, where

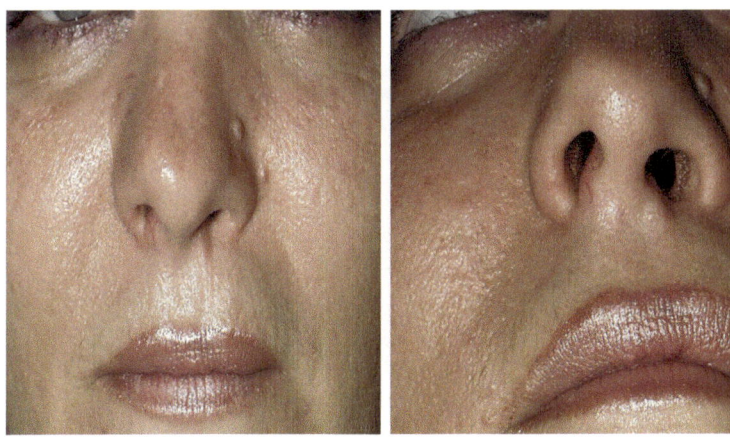

Figure 7.3 Undiagnosed left unilateral cleft lip.

Adult female with a clinically, subtle cleft lip. Left – the visible line along the left philtral column is evidence of an underlying separation of the lip muscle (i.e., the orbicularis muscle, OO). Right – nostril asymmetry, another subtle sign of the left cleft lip. This patient presented with her daughter who had an obvious cleft lift with complete separation of the lip. She had never realized that she also was born with a cleft.

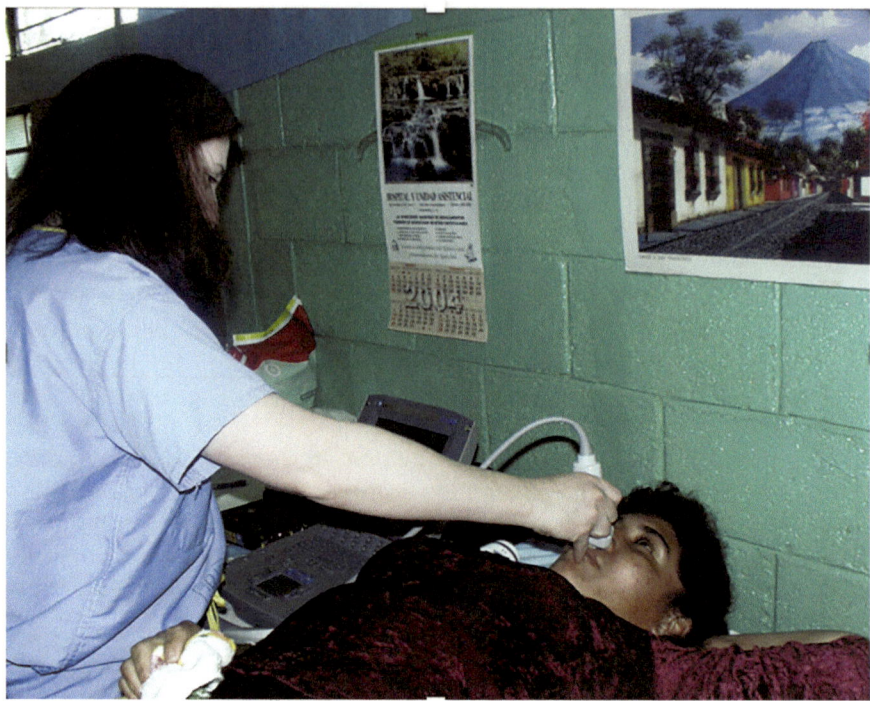

Figure 7.4 Study design to check for subclinical discontinuity of the Orbicularis Oris Muscle (OOM) in family members of patients with an obvious cleft lip.

The upper lip of each family member was scanned with an Ultrasound (US) to check for defects in the OOM. Defects would indicate the presence of subclinical cleft lip (image taken during a Plastic Surgery Mission Trip to Guatemala).

I knew surgeons from my previous fellowship in Spain, and screened an additional 144 children and family members in 3 days. Over the years the non-overt signs of clefting for which we screened expanded to include 3D pictures of the face, speech samples, olfaction, and dental anomalies. We correlated and validated the ultrasound finding with cadaver dissections.[10] In 2010 at the Children's Hospital of Colorado, 82 additional participants were screened over a 2-day weekend from the Cleft Program. The productivity of these research blitzes has been tremendous; as of this writing, well over 30 manuscripts have been published using the data from Guatemala, Madrid, and/or Colorado. Multiple new genes have been identified that are associated with an increased risk of clefting.[11] Genetic counseling has been improved and refined. Patients and family members are now routinely screened for more subtle signs of a cleft defect, such as abnormalities in speech and facial asymmetries.

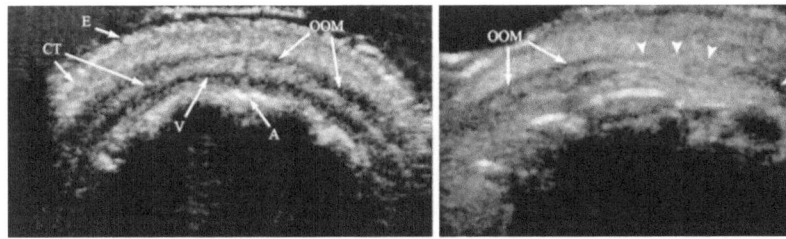

Figure 7.5 Ultrasound of a normal lip (left), and one with defects in the OOM (right).

In an ultrasound image the **OOM** is represented as a hypoechogenic (dark) band. In contrast, the skin (**E**) and connective tissue (**CT**) are echogenic bright. Discontinuities (i.e., defects) of the **OOM** are seen as localized echogenic (light) areas within the hypoechogenic muscle tissue (labelled with white arrowheads). **V** = Vestibule (i.e., the space between the lips and gums and teeth). **A** = Alveolar ridge. [Reprinted from **Anatomical Basis for Apparent Subepithelial Cleft Lip: A histological and Ultrasonographic Survey of the Orbicularis Oris Muscle (Fig. 1a, p. 521; Fig 2a, p. 523) by Carolyn Rogers, Seth Weinberg, Timothy Smith, Frederic White-Brown Deleyiannis, Mark Mooney, Mary Marazita.** *Cleft Palate Craniofac* J 2008. (**Copyright Sage Publishing, 2008**)].

The personal rewards of doing clinical and basic science research can be extremely satisfying. There is a somewhat selfish thrill in describing or discovering something new, in demonstrating that your surgical technique is an improvement compared to other techniques. Your research can improve patient care, provide confidence that you are offering a well-thought-out treatment plan, and make you a better surgeon by challenging yourself. However, there are certain financial facts, opportunity costs, about research that every surgeon must consider.

The American health care system rewards productivity, not necessarily quality. Surgeons are directly reimbursed according to how much they bill, by how many procedures they do; not by how well they perform the procedures, nor by how well their patients do. Every hour spent doing research is an hour not doing surgery, not billing. Surgeons in private practice experience this reality most acutely. It simply cannot be possible to financially support your staff and cover the costs of running a practice if you devote a considerable amount of time doing research and not operating.

The majority of clinical research is done by academic surgeons employed at universities or by surgeons employed within a large health system. Salaries are typically guaranteed at some minimum level. Incentives based on other metrics, such as clinical volume (i.e., patients seen, operations done, work RVUs), papers published, or grant money awarded, can advance one's compensation above this minimum. However, "you should not have gone into academics if you wanted to make money" is an often-repeated comment. This has been said to me and likely to the majority of surgeons at some point in their careers. Usually, this comment is initiated by the Chief of the Department or of the Surgical Division. The statement is somewhat hypocritical, since it often originates from those who are paid the most by the university or the health system and from those for whom clinical productivity is often not demanded or expected. However, it is not an unfair statement. Surgeons in leadership have achieved these positions through hard work and their efforts to obtain a national reputation, usually based on research.

What remains the challenge is how to fairly compensate all of the members of a Surgical Division, not just the Chief, when there is a diverse faculty with varying interests in and commitments to clinical medicine, research, and teaching. Contemporary academic programs are not significantly different from nonacademic programs or private groups. For both, clinical revenue dictates solvency.

For plastic surgeons, there are three main avenues of obtaining grant support: through the National Institutes of Health (NIH); the Plastic Surgery Foundation (PSF); and local institutional support, such as from your university. The NIH offers dozens of types of grants. The Research Project Grant, or RO1 grant, has the longest history and is considered the most prestigious. All small grants, such as those from the PSF or from your university, are expected or awarded with the aspiration of leading to a larger NIH grant. R01 grants support a "discrete, specified, circumscribed" project and are expected to produce results that are specific and actionable. They typically are awarded for 3 to 5 years with annual budgets of approximately $400,000–$500,000. These grants are extremely competitive, with only approximately 10% of applications being funded. Two to 3 months of dedicated time are required just to write the grant application. According to the most recent survey of all academic plastic surgeons at 94 programs, published in 2016, only 18 investigators (2.1%) were NIH funded at 12 programs (12.8%).[12] Seventy-seven percent of these grants were awarded through the RO1 mechanism.

Congress has legislatively mandated a limitation on the direct salary for individuals awarded NIH grants. In 2024 the salary cap for the full-time leader of the research (i.e., Principal Investigator, [PI]) of an RO1 is $221,900 per year. If only 50% of the PI's time is devoted to research, then the salary limitation is $110,950 per year. The disparity between this salary cap and the compensation paid to a clinical active plastic surgeon can be a major barrier to research. Consider that this difference is more than twofold when comparing it to the median total compensation of an Assistant Professor of Plastic Surgery ($444,599, according to the 2024 Medical Group Management Association Compensation survey).[13] This disparity widens with increasing academic rank. Moreover, compared to the median compensation of a plastic surgeon in private practice, the difference widens even further.

If a plastic surgeon wishes to pursue research, they must make a conscious financial choice. One will likely need to limit clinical time to create time for research. Importantly, one must be at peace with the realization that your compensation will likely not reach the level of your peers who only treat patients. Medical school graduates now owe a median average of $200,000 to $215,000 in total educational debt.[14] One must consider this debt in any long-term financial and professional plan. Additionally, if you are in a program which taxes the clinical revenue generated by the group to support research, one must realize that your compensation will be shifted to support those doing more research and less clinical work.

The ultimate purpose of research is to give back, to share what you have learned. Surgery has a much more lasting effect, both for your patients and personally, if combined with clinical research. Developmental psychologist Erik Erikson (1902–1994) had this great quote: "I am what survives of me". That is really quite a different sort of motivation compared to ambitions about finances or improvements in your work-life balance. It requires a real conscious decision to step out of the moment to think about oneself in a chain of influence. You have to decide what sort of legacy you wish to leave for posterity. Your legacy should be a labor of love – not a chore. If you do not love doing research, then leave it, but ask yourself how you can support those that do. All too often medicine has become fragmented by people trying to serve their own needs and short-term loyalties. Your needs and motivations will change as you enter different phases of your surgical career. Direct involvement or indirect support of clinical research offers one way to unify surgeons and to help patients beyond a daily encounter.

There is always something to look at and improve, if you just open your eyes.

REFERENCES

1. Tavernise S. The new smoke: a hot debate over e-cigarettes as a path to tobacco, or from it. *The New York Times*, February 22, 2014 (https://nytimes.com/2014/02/23/health/a-hot-debate-over-e-cigarettes-as-a-path-to-tobacco-or-from-it.html).
2. Doll R, Hill AB. Smoking and carcinoma of the lung. *BMJ* 1950;221(2):739–748.
3. Doll R, Peto R, Boreham J, Sutherland I. Mortality in relation to smoking: 50 years' observations on male British doctors. *BMJ*. 2004 June 26; 328(7455):1519.
4. Feinstein AR. The pre-therapeutic classification of co-morbidity in chronic disease. *J Chron Dis* 1973;23:455–469.
5. Deleyiannis FW-B, Thomas DB, Vaughn TL, Davis S. Alcoholism: Independent predictor of survival in patients with head and neck cancer. *J Natl Cancer Inst* 1996; 88:542–549.
6. Rau A, Reinikovaite V, Schmidt E, Taraseviciene-Stewart L, Deleyiannis FW-B. Electronic cigarettes are as toxic to skin flap survival as tobacco cigarettes. *Ann Plas Surg*. 2017 Jul;79(1):86–91.
7. Reinikovaite V, Rodriguez IE, Karoor V, Rau A, Trinh BB, Deleyiannis FW-B, Taraseviciene-Stewart L. The effects of electronic cigarette vapor on the lung: direct comparison to tobacco smoke. *Eur Respir J*. 2018 Apr 4;51(4):1701661.

8. Weinberg SM, Neiswanger K, Martin RA, Mooney MP, Kane AA, Wenger SL, Losee J, Deleyiannis F, Ma L, De Salamanca JE, Czeizel AE, Marazita ML. The Pittsburgh Oral-Facial Cleft Study: expanding the cleft phenotype. Background and justification. *Cleft Palate Craniofac J.* 2006 Jan;43(1):7-20.

9. Neiswanger K, Deleyiannis FW, Avila JR, Cooper ME, Brandon CA, Vieira AR, Noorchashm N, Weinberg SM, Bardi KM, Murray JC, Marazita ML. Candidate genes for oral-facial clefts in Guatemalan families. *Ann Plast Surg.* 2006 May;56(5):518–521; discussion 521.

10. Roger CR, Weinberg SM, Smith TD, Deleyiannis FWB, Mooney MP, Marazita ML. Anatomical basis for apparent subepithelial cleft lip: A histological and ultrasonographic survey of the orbicularis oris muscle. *Cleft Palate Craniofac J* 2008 Sept;45(5):518–524.

11. Indencleef K, Hoskens H, Lee MK, White JD, Liu C, Eller RJ, Naqvi S, Wehby GL, Moreno Uribe LM, Hecht JT, Long RE Jr, Christensen K, Deleyiannis FW, Walsh S, Shriver MD, Richmond S, Wysocka J, Peeters H, Shaffer JR, Marazita ML, Hens G, Weinberg SM, Claes P. The intersection of the genetic architecture of orofacial clefts and normal facial variation. *Front Genet.* 2021 Feb 22;12:626403.

12. Silvestre J, Abbatematteo JM, Serletti J, Chang B. National Institutes of Health funding in plastic surgery: a crisis? *Plast Reconstr Surg* 2016 138(3):732–739.

13. Medical Group Management Association – MGMA. 2024 provider compensation data report. Academic compensation. Total compensation by faculty rank. Data extracted from MGMA DataDrive, July 16, 2024.

14. Hanson M. Average medical school debt, EducationalData.org, November 22, 2022 (https://educationaldata.org/average-medical-school-debt).

Chapter 8

Takeaways for the patient undergoing reconstruction

> Never tell a patient that you can fix them. You cannot. You can only help them recover. They will never be exactly the same.
>
> – Doug Newton, MD, 1942–2018
> *Pittsburgh microsurgeon, plastic surgeon,*
> *and mentor to a generation of plastic surgeons*

Every patient who suffers a major trauma or cancer will be transformed. The event, the diagnosis, and the subsequent treatment(s) will be life-altering. How can one acquire hope, skills, and knowledge so that this transformation becomes positive? How can we modify our behaviors and decision-making capabilities to make these improvements?

This chapter will summarize some of the principal observations and recommendations that may help patients as they undergo reconstruction. The following themes will be summarized: (1) access to microsurgical expertise; (2) recognition that physical and psychological healing may never be complete, but that there are tools that can influence how you feel; (3) awareness that the resilience and grit may be the best predictors of how to overcome a disability; (4) communication with your surgeon, particularly in creating a conversation about the goals, benefits, and risks of the reconstruction that is being proposed; and (5) legacy options for the patient wishing to help others going through a similar experience.

IS MICROSURGERY (I.E., FREE TISSUE TRANSFER) AN OPTION FOR YOUR RECONSTRUCTION?

Microsurgery is transplant surgery using tissue from your own body. If you have lost a piece of tissue (i.e., skin, muscle, and/or bone) from trauma or cancer, it can likely be replaced with another piece of tissue from your body. This requires detaching the blood supply of this tissue and transferring the undamaged tissue to the site of the defect, of the trauma or cancer. The tissue is made "free" (i.e., momentarily without any perfusion or connection to the body). The blood supply of the transferred tissue must be reattached to

DOI: 10.1201/9781003538028-9

vessels around the site of the defect. This is typically done with an operating microscope because the vessels are so small (i.e., 1–3 mm). The tissue is cut, sewn, and shaped into the form and function of the missing tissue.

Free tissue transfer has been available only since the 1970s. It has revolutionized how cancer and trauma patients are treated. Almost any defect can potentially be reconstructed with a free flap if the surgical expertise is available. Ask your treatment team about this option. At the very least, it may initiate the first conversation and consultation with a reconstructive surgeon who can discuss multiple possibilities for reconstruction.

IS RECONSTRUCTION YOUR PRIORITY?

The goals of reconstruction are to improve function and/or appearance (i.e., quality of life), but in the short term, reconstruction can mean more operations, more time in the hospital, more time away from your job and family, and maybe more acute pain. Can you envision living without an extremity, without a breast, without the body part that has been injured? Almost all defects of the face and head and neck require reconstruction because function and appearance will be affected too profoundly. However, it is not uncommon for women with breast cancer to decide to not undergo reconstruction. Numerous surveys report that about 50%–60% of women who undergo a complete mastectomy (i.e., removal of the entire breast) do not receive any type of breast reconstruction. It is unknown how access, cost, and personal choice each uniquely and independently affects this overall percentage. However, certainly one of the main reasons is that many patients may wish to focus on beating the cancer. Reconstruction becomes a secondary priority, and it can often be successfully done after the cancer has been beaten.

In every major hospital and medical center in the United States, newly diagnosed breast cancer patients are discussed at multidisciplinary breast cancer tumor boards that are typically accredited by the National Accreditation Program for Breast Centers (NAPBC). Part of the NAPBC's standards is the expectation/goal that 100% of patients are educated about reconstructive options. More specifically, "as part of the informed decision-making process, every effort should be made to ensure patients undergoing a mastectomy are offered a pre-operative discussion with a reconstructive/Plastic Surgeon".[1] Assuming this goal is being met (which is questionable), still, only a minority of patients may receive reconstruction even after talking with a plastic surgeon.

A leg mangled by trauma is routinely amputated in medical facilities that do not have access to microsurgical expertise. In the developing world, this scenario occurs in the majority of hospitals. Volunteer for a medical mission trip that includes a prosthetist/orthotist, and you will be overwhelmed by the sheer number of amputees who come to receive a possible limb prosthetic. An amputation is a quick and technically easy operation that allows a patient to leave the hospital and to begin to heal. The most common type of amputation after trauma is a below the knee amputation. With the right prosthetic device, physical rehabilitation, and the right mindset, amputees can have a significant improvement in their quality of life.

Unlike breast reconstruction, the government does not mandate that insurance companies cover prostheses. However, most marketplace (i.e., HMO-based) and government (i.e., Medicare and Medicaid) insurance will provide some or near-complete coverage. Insurance coverage will vary based on carrier, type of prosthesis, prior authorization, type of facility, and whether the doctor or prosthetist/orthotist/prosthodontists accepts the assignment. Head and neck reconstruction with free tissue transfer will routinely be covered by all insurance.

IS THERE ACCESS TO MICROSURGICAL EXPERTISE IN YOUR TREATING FACILITY?

In general, microsurgical expertise is provided by surgeons who have focused their practice on microsurgery. These surgeons are board-certified by the American Board of Plastic Surgery and/or the American Board of Otolaryngology – Head and Neck Surgery (Oto-HNS). This is a distinct minority in both specialties, and usually these surgeons are not marketing themselves as cosmetic surgeons. They are reconstructive surgeons. They will also likely be well-educated in cosmetic surgery, but it will likely not be their preferred practice.

Microsurgeons board-certified only in Oto-HNS will focus their practice on patients requiring reconstruction of the face, mouth, throat, and head. They will likely also be fellowship trained in treating head and neck oncology patients. Microsurgeons board-certified only in plastic surgery tend to focus their practice on breast reconstruction. Some will also do limb reconstruction. Every facility, academic and nonacademic, especially if they are treating trauma and complex cancer patients, should have a few surgeons that have expertise in microsurgery. The experience and training of these surgeons will likely vary greatly from those having multiple board certifications and fellowship training to those who do just a few microsurgical cases a year. You, the patient, should not hesitate about asking your surgeon about his/her experience, training, and expertise.

Access to breast microsurgical reconstruction (i.e., DIEP flaps) is perhaps the hardest to understand. Recent news reports, echoing patient advocacy group and plastic surgeons, have stressed that plastic surgeons may stop offering women with private insurance DIEP flap reconstruction if the S codes which are billed to insurance are recoded to a lower-paying CPT code.[2,3] This is true. Presently, many Plastic surgeons will not see a patient for DIEP reconstruction unless the insurance is private and pays well. The reality is that S codes pay the surgeon much more than other microsurgical

CPT codes, even though many other types of free flaps may require more work, a longer hospital stay, and broader experience. At larger health care facilities, especially academic facilities and those that employ plastic surgeons, this should not be of much concern. Patients will likely not be turned away if they have government insurance or poor-paying insurance. Also, there is no reason to assume that the care you receive will be inferior. In fact, the surgeons at these facilities are often busier and more experienced than those focusing just on patients with high-paying insurance.

WHY IS IT IMPORTANT TO UNDERSTAND THE STAGES OF GRIEF?

Grief is a natural emotion that occurs when one goes through a loss. Death, divorce, and any major change in life, such as those caused by trauma and a cancer diagnosis, can cause one to grieve. In 1969, American Swiss psychiatrist Elisabeth Kubler-Ross in her book *On Death and Dying* originally described the emotional suffering of grief to occur in five stages: denial, anger, bargaining, depression, and acceptance.[4] Whether everyone goes through these five stages, either completely or sequentially, is debatable, but they are important to understand so one can anticipate and comprehend what he/she is feeling and hopefully adapt and accept the change. Grieving takes time.

Denial is the initial defense mechanism that one uses to protect oneself from the reality of the loss. It helps you survive the loss. You think losing a leg, a breast, or a piece of your face has no meaning. It is overwhelming; you may go numb. Denial gives your brain time to process and recognize what has happened.

Anger is a natural way of expressing pain. The loss of a body part will likely seem cruel and unfair. Anger at the disease, those involved in the accident, or the circumstances that lead to the event gives some temporary structure to the meaninglessness of the loss. It is normal to want to feel angry rather than helpless.

Bargaining is a way to regain control. It is natural to want to feel like you can affect the outcome. You create a lot of "what if" or "only if" statements. These statements may be verbalized or internal and could be medical, religious, or social. Bargaining is often a sign the loss has been conceded, but it is also a way to hang onto hope.

Depression, or acute sadness, is when the loss of the body part profoundly affects your life, your ability for enjoyment, interactions with family and others, and likely employment. This can be the longest stage of grief. Depression can also manifest as irritability. To cope with this sadness and/or irritability, one should seek support from family and friends and see a psychiatrist for an evaluation. Cognitive therapy and medications can significantly help.

Acceptance means that you accept the new reality of your loss. It does not mean that your grief is over; the body part will always be missing. Acceptance means that you are healing and that you realize that there are more good days to come. Your thoughts and behavior will likely become future orientated.

THE FEAR OF DEATH AND YOUR "LIFE SENTENCE"

Trauma or a cancer diagnosis will cause the fear of death to directly invade into your life. Most people when considering death will try to reduce this fear by challenging the possibility that it will happen any time soon. However, as a patient who has just been diagnosed with cancer or gone through a traumatic event, this fear might be quite acute, overwhelming, and very real. Confronting and accepting this awareness of death can become a profound way to find new purpose and meaning in life. This does not mean giving up on life; on the contrary, hopefully it triggers one to pay more attention to those values and persons that provide meaning. This may be the event that moves one to articulate (perhaps even write down) the "life sentence" that outlines how you want to be remembered.

HOW TO CREATE A LIFE WITH MEANING

The most important thing in life is to be of service to other people, to orient your actions and path toward helping others. The patients in this book, as well as the many others whom I have treated, who seem to do the best, are those who step outside themselves to a greater purpose. This has been as simple as focusing or spending more time with family or friends, or as complex as becoming a national/regional advocate for a particular cause, such as promoting greater access to health care. To reorient one's focus or direction, one should start with small changes and keep them consistent. Slow change is sustainable change.

Children have a remarkable ability to see what is good and meaningful. They will often want to help others as they have been helped. This message of slow, consistent change can be extremely impactful to children and young adults as they look decades ahead to their life after trauma or cancer. To consciously create an opportunity for yourself where you can be in a position to provide unique help, one should be prepared for an enormous commitment. This means becoming aware of the sequential small steps that one has to walk before any long-term goal is reached.

In this book I have tried to describe the education and experience needed to become a microsurgeon. Seeing the remarkable, life-changing results of reconstruction is inspiring. Viewing these successes, more than a few medical students and residents have told me that it is their desire to become a microsurgeon. However, it is the small steps that typically convince many to pursue other medical specialties. Comments and exclamations that I and other microsurgeons have heard include: "Oh my gosh, you spent nearly 10 years after medical school training as a surgeon before you were an attending!", and "that operation took 9 hours; how can you do that every week?". Years of formal education, hours and hours in the operating room, and a gradual awareness of your abilities (mentally and physically) are the small steps. Success is the end result of long-term practice and perseverance.

As patients look to create a life with meaning, it is the small steps that one should plan. Becoming a microsurgeon is an extreme example of the thousands of steps one must walk before reaching a goal. However, to be successful in any endeavor, especially in those that will positively help others, you need to build an ability to step back from your thoughts and observe them. More succinctly, you need to be mindful of how your present actions or plans will be connected to what is good and meaningful. As a reality, this is easy to say, and much harder to do.

Something that I began to appreciate only after listening to the stories of recovery of my own patients is the value of meditation. This small step, often only 10 minutes a day listening to a mediation app, can help reduce stress and regulate emotion. With mindfulness meditation, one can practice paying attention to the present moment and observe sensations and emotions as they come and go without getting caught up or overwhelmed by them. Perhaps the biggest advantage of meditation is that it formally allows one to intentionally focus on those emotions that will help produce a hopeful and positive future. Meditation enables one to influence how he/she feels. For patients suffering from anxiety and pain after surgery, mediation can be a useful tool.

THE GRIT FACTOR IN RECOVERY AFTER RECONSTRUCTION

According to psychologist Angela Duckworth, grit is a combination of passion and long-term perseverance that leads to achievement.[5] She states,

> many of us, it seems, quit what we start far too early and far too often. Even more than the effort a gritty person puts in on a single day, what matters is that they wake up the next day, and the next day, ready to get on that treadmill and keep going.[5]

To be successful, one needs to live life as if running a marathon, not a sprint.

After a life-altering surgery, recovery requires a deliberate, sustained effort. This effort will likely involve seeking out therapy (physical and psychological), developing networks of assistance (possibly with doctors, career counselors, and social workers) and coping strategies (especially for stress), and trying to find mentors who have successfully recovered from a similar experience. With a support network of friends, family, and mentors, a person can develop grit and build the resilience to keep moving forward.

Other than surrounding oneself with positive and supportive mentors and friends, one must plan and make deliberate practice a habit. Angela Duckworth lists the basic requirements of deliberate practice:

- A clearly defined stretch goal
- Full concentration and effort
- Immediate and informative feedback
- Repetition with reflection and refinement

After facial trauma and treatment for extensive cancers of the face, head, and /or neck, outward appearance and daily functions, such as eating and talking, may be affected; for breast cancer, body image, sexuality, and intimacy; for limb salvage, the ability to walk and to participate in activities that require independent mobility. For a patient recovering from these diagnoses or treatments, goals will likely initially focus on what has been lost. Reconstruction can certainly improve many of these functions. However, some function and emotional well-being may never be fully regained, even with the hardest or most diligent practice. What seems to pull patients out of perseverating on this loss, out of the grief, is a reprioritization of what is important in their lives. They focus on what is left. With this reprioritization, new goals (not focused on lost) are then set, plans are made, and hope is restored. Multiple support groups, such as Support for People with Oral and Head and Neck Cancer (SPOHNC),[6] the National Breast Cancer Foundation Support Group,[7] and the Amputee Coalition,[8] are available to help persons obtain feedback and reflect on the way forward.

BALANCED DISCUSSION WITH YOUR SURGEON

A balanced discussion means telling your surgeon what your priorities may be, and the surgeon willing to be honest about what he/she can reliably deliver to meet these priorities. The conversation is always gray with nuances of benefit and risk.

Surgeons cannot predict how someone will cope with a life-altering event. However, when patients have obvious family involvement, grit, and a mindset oriented toward the future, we may more likely recommend an "aggressive reconstruction" (i.e., limb salvage versus amputation, DIEP flap versus no breast reconstruction). "Aggressive" is a term used by surgeons and patients alike to describe a procedure that may seem more complicated, invasive, and potentially riskier than an alternative. The surgery is invasive, but it is not destructive. It is offered as a constructive means to meet the patient's long-term goals.

If we believe that the long-term benefits of reconstruction outweigh the short-term disadvantages (i.e., longer hospital stay, more acute pain), we will likely recommend a more "aggressive" treatment. This is particularly true if we sense that the patient has family support and a mindset that will assist them during this process. Thus, any discussion about reconstruction should focus not just on what to expect in the short term (i.e., until you are physically healed, usually by 6 weeks), but importantly on how the proposed procedure may offer benefits for the rest of your life.

Most patients and even most doctors, unless they are microsurgeons, will likely not have the medical experience to know if a free flap will be needed. "Is a free flap a better option?" is typically the right question. For a surgeon to answer this question comprehensively, they must do microsurgery – more to the point, a lot of microsurgery (i.e., every week, every month). Otherwise, to paraphrase Sir William Osler (1849–1919), founding Professor of Johns Hopkins Hospital, "their recommendations have not been learned at the bedside".[9]

CREATING A LONG-LASTING IMPACT

Talking with someone who has gone through a similar experience with cancer, trauma, and /or reconstruction can provide a patient with hope and comfort. Being available to talk to other patients, either informally by phone, more regularly in established support groups, or more widespread by doing regional or national interviews, is a direct way to help others and pass on those lessons that you believe create meaning.

Giving financially to institutions has a beneficial role, but what seems to have the most long-lasting, personal reward are those commitments that require stewardship. This means careful and responsible management of a cause, particularly of the resources that you have established and given to support that cause. An institution/university can likely develop and provide meaningful services and programs with your gift. However, when financial gifts are given to institutions or universities, you, the donor, often lose some of the ability to be the steward. Continual involvement, in the purpose and the direction of your gift, will potentially involve the setting up of your own nonprofit organization (NPO).

An NPO provides a way for you to bring people together for a common goal to shape actions. A NPO qualifies for tax-exempt status by the IRS because its mission is to provide a public benefit. To become a nonprofit, one must apply for 501(c)(3) status to the IRS. A nonprofit pays no taxes on any money received through fundraising.

As founders or members of NPOs, some of my patients and their family members have been able to direct the purpose of their giving and, importantly, the results. As an example, the John Lester Foundation (JFL) was founded in 2016 as an NPO.[10] According to the mission statement,

"Our vision is a world where all children are aware of reconstructive treatment options, have access to these life changing operations and receive the absolute best in care regardless of financial situation or location". Since its founding, over $750,000 dollars have been raised, and hundreds of children have received free medical and surgical care. The JFL has created a legacy of hope and giving for all those involved.

For patients considering how best to establish their own legacy, there are multiple options. Personal time devoted to talking to others suffering a similar health crisis, financial contributions, and the establishment of an NPO are all wonderful opportunities. However, the sharing of realistic optimism is perhaps the most unseen gift. From a patient's perspective, it means accepting what you can and cannot control. You cannot control your cancer diagnosis or the trauma that has placed you in the hospital, but you can control how much effort you put into your recovery. Other people, whether it be family, other patients, friends, and/or clinicians, are always watching. Your efforts will likely inspire others in ways that you will never know.

REFERENCES

1. American College of Surgeons. *National Accreditation Program for Breast Centers Standards Manual*, 2018 edition, p. 54.
2. American Society of Plastic Surgeons. *Press Release. Survey: Many U.S. Women Lack Basic Information on Life After Mastectomy*. Study Finds Many Women Simply Don't Know About Concerns Ranging From Breast Sensation to Insurance Coverage for Breast Reconstruction. October 17, 2022.
3. Werner A, Winick LA, Pradhan R. How a medical recoding may limit patient's options for breast reconstruction. *CBS Mornings*, May 31, 2023.
4. Kubler-Ross E. *On Death and Dying*. Macmillan, 1969.
5. Duckworth A. *Grit: the power of passion and perseverance*. Scribner, 2016.
6. Support for People with Oral and Head and Neck Cancer, Inc. (SPOHNC) (https://spohnc.org).
7. National Breast Cancer Foundation, Inc., Breast Cancer Support Group (https://www.nationalbreastcancer.org).
8. Amputee Coalition (https://www.amoutee-coalition.org).
9. Thayer WS. Osler the teacher. *Johns Hopkins Hospital Bulletin* 1919: v. 30, p. 198.
10. The John Lester Foundation (https://www.johnlesterfoundation.org).

In memoriam
Mary Taylor Deleyiannis (1941–2024)

To my mom, who in her artwork inspired her children and grandchildren to try consciously to create what we could imagine.

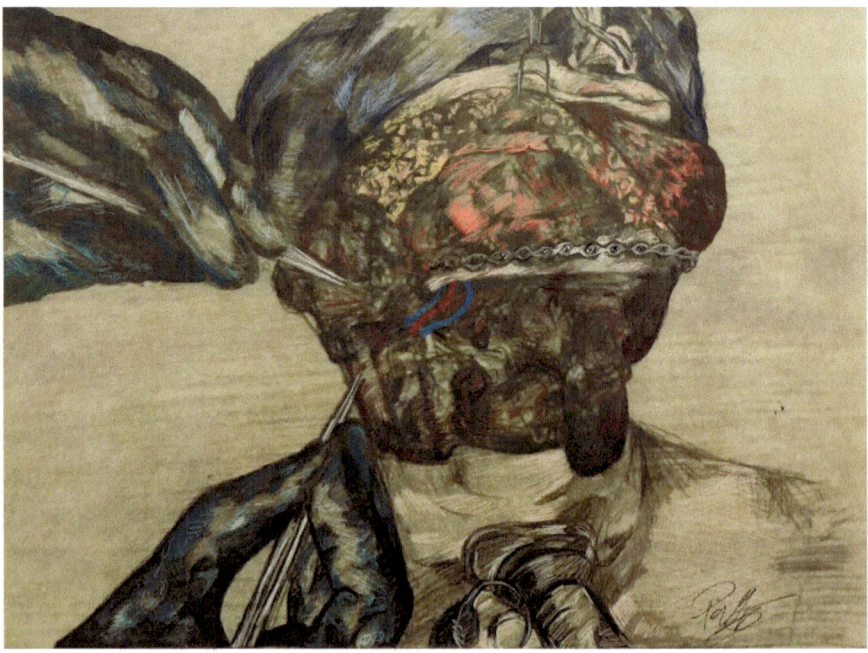

Mandible reconstruction with a fibular free flap (Artist: Paloma Deleyiannis). Sketch the operation before the first cut. You will likely see options that you have not yet considered.

DOI: 10.1201/9781003538028-10

Index

Pages in *italics* refer to figures.